HEADACHES
& MIGRAINE

A SELF-HELP GUIDE

COMBINING ORTHODOX AND COMPLEMENTARY APPROACHES TO HEALTH

HEADWAY HEALTHWISE

HEADACHES & MIGRAINE

A SELF-HELP GUIDE ·
COMBINING ORTHODOX AND COMPLEMENTARY APPROACHES TO HEALTH

HASNAIN WALJI & DR ANDREA KINGSTON

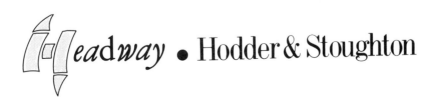

Headway • Hodder & Stoughton

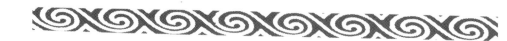

Cataloguing in Publication Data is available from the British Library

ISBN 0 340 60560 X

First published 1994
Impression number   10   9   8   7   6   5   4   3   2   1
Year   1998   1997   1996   1995   1994

Printed in Great Britain for Hodder & Stoughton Educational, a division of Hodder Headline Plc, 338 Euston Road, London NW1 3BH by Page Bros (Norwich) Ltd.

CONTENTS

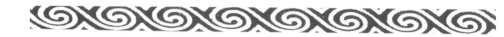

*This book is dedicated to the seekers of health
and to those who help them find it.*

ACKNOWLEDGEMENTS

I should like to express my gratitude to Dr Andrea Kingston for her valuable input and the enlightened way she dealt with a number of apparent contradictions between orthodox medicine and complementary therapies; to nutritionist Angela Dowden for offering many pertinent suggestions; to Sato Liu of the Natural Medicines Society for her assistance in providing contacts and arranging interviews with practitioners; and to my agent Susan Mears for her encouragement and practical help.

This book could not possibly have been written without the co-operation of the following practitioners who have so willingly endured my interruptions: aromatherapy – Christine Wildwood; naturopathy – Jan De Vries; homoeopathy – Michael Thompson and Beth MacEoin; reflexology – Pauline Wills; and anthroposophical medicine – Dr Maurice Orange.

I must thank my daughter Sukaina for giving her time during vacation from university for wading through research papers and books and extracting relevant information. Last but not least, I wish to thank my wife Latifa whose gentle care and concern, not to mention long hours typing the manuscript, enabled me to complete this book.

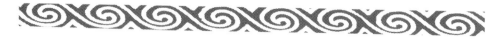

Foreword To The Series
from the Natural Medicines Society

When we visit our doctor's surgery and are given a diagnosis, we often receive a prescription at the same time. More people than ever are now aware that there may be complementary treatments available and would like to explore the possibilities, but do not know which kind of treatment would be most useful for their problem.

There are books on just about every treatment available, but few which start from this standpoint: the patient interested in knowing the options for treating their particular condition – which treatment is available or useful, what the treatment involves, or what to expect when consulting the practitioner.

The Headway Healthwise series will provide the answers for those wishing to consider what treatment is available, once the doctor has diagnosed their condition. Each book will cover both the orthodox and complementary approaches. Although patients are naturally most interested in relieving their immediate symptoms, the books show how complementary treatment goes much deeper; underlying causes are explored and the patient is treated as a whole.

It is important to stress that it is not the intention of this series to replace the expertise of the doctors and practitioners, nor to encourage self-treatment, but to show the options available to the patient.

As the consumer charity working for freedom of choice in medicine, the Natural Medicines Society welcomes the Headway Healthwise series. Although the Natural Medicines Society does not recommend people who are taking prescribed orthodox medicines to stop doing so, our aim is to introduce them to complementary forms of treatment. We believe the orthodox system of medicine is often best used as a last, not first, resort when other, gentler, methods fail or are inappropriate.

Giving patients the information to make their choice is the purpose of this series. With the increasing use of complementary medicine within the NHS, knowing the complementary options is vital both to the patients and to their doctors in the search for better health care.

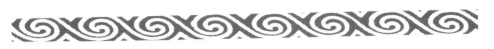

Foreword To The Book

Migraine is one of the most common ailments of man and an illness of great antiquity, having been described by Hippocrates (400BC) and Avicenna (980-1037AD). It is believed that something of the order of one in ten people suffer from migraine to some extent. However, its severity and the frequency of attacks varies widely from the occasional mild headache to severe, incapacitating attacks which occur frequently.

People in this last group were those I saw most often in my years consulting at the Migraine Clinic of the Royal London Homoeopathic Hospital (sadly, now defunct). Certainly, those suffering so severely are well advised to see a specialist practitioner from one of the medical disciplines described in this book.

Likewise, those who have been struggling on for years, and these are the majority of sufferers, may well find help from some of the treatments and approaches described here. I am very aware from my own experience that many of these patients do not see their General Practitioners, either from fear of an unsympathetic reception or because they have found prescribed treatments unhelpful, or productive of side-effects.

It is in fact remarkable that the vast amount of research in orthodox medicine into migraine has produced so little in the way of treatments, or reasons for its occurrence. It is for this reason, among others, that The Natural Medicines Society is endorsing *Headaches and Migraine.* The Society also hopes that those who read this book, and, hopefully, benefit from the treatments described, will join the NMS (membership is open to everybody), which needs support both to defend the position of natural medicines in a hostile world and to promote research into the use and development of these medicines.

Headaches are far less debilitating than migraine but affect almost everyone at some time in their lives; by being informed about the different types of headaches and their possible causes and triggers, and by being aware of the appropriate natural medicines and complementary therapies available, sufferers can take steps to both reduce the frequency and lessen the severity of attacks.

It is an interesting but little known fact that currently more than half the world's population are dependent on natural medicines for treatment of their illnesses. Hence the importance of research in

this area and the preservation of the plant species of known or potential medical use. It is clear, therefore, that the preservation and development of natural medicines is not merely of national but of international importance, not only in the treatment of headaches and migraine, but for medicine in general.

Dr Geoffrey Douch
GP specialising in homoeopathic & anthroposophical medicine
Member of the Natural Medicines Society Council and its
Medicines Advisory Research Committee

PREFACE

Headway Healthwise is a concise new series which takes the original approach of looking at common ailments and describing how they may be treated using complementary therapies. The aim of the series is not to replace the orthodox medical approach but to give readers an overview of how they may be helped by consulting complementary practitioners.

Once a condition has been diagonised by a GP, those wishing to avail themselves of other forms of treatment will find this book particularly useful. The intention of this series is not to recommend people taking prescribed orthodox medicines to stop taking these. It is to introduce them to alternative and complementary forms of treatment which may enable them reduce the amount of orthodox prescriptions at the very least and in many cases do away with their need altogether.

We have attempted to present the information in a style that is clear and easy to read. The central approach is to look at headaches and migraine from different perspectives by providing you with descriptions of several complementary therapies. While cautioning against self-medication, the book has been written to encourage you to take charge of your own health by making an informed choice of therapy. It shows how and why orthodox medicine – a life-saving and useful system of medicine – should be used as a last resort when other more natural methods fail, rather than the first recourse.

An overview of headaches and migraine in the opening chapter is followed by a chapter on the kind of treatment to expect from your GP. The third chapter deals with such factors as lifestyle, diet and nutrition in the management of these disorders. Later chapters look at complementary approaches.

The one common factor that underpins all the alternative or complementary therapeutic techniques described in this book is the belief in the healing power of the body. Practitioners recognise that the body possesses an inherent ability to cure itself. This gives a clear message to the patient of his/her role in the healing process – that of the mind willing the body to heal itself.

At first sight this may appear to challenge the approach of orthodox medicine, in which the therapeutic objective is to cure the diseased part of the body. The patient has no role to play except dutifully to take the medicine. The concept of a white-coated god who possesses the magic pill to cure is the result of fear combined

with a lack of understanding of the nature of disease and, more so, that of health.

This book is an attempt to dispel the myths and to bring about a greater understanding of the issues relating to health and healing, which go beyond the realms of simple anatomy and biology. The recognition that orthodox medicine and complementary therapies need not be mutually exclusive, as both have a role to play, can go a long way towards promoting the integrated medicine of the twenty-first century.

Hasnain Walji
Milton Keynes
January, 1994

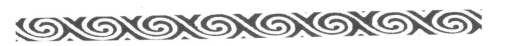

Note: Any information given in this book is not intended to be taken as a replacement for medical advice. Any person with a condition requiring medical attention should consult a medical professional.

Throughout the book you will find some words in italics. If these are not immediately explained, you will find the explanation in the glossary.

1

OVERVIEW: IT'S JUST A HEADACHE – OR IS IT?

Headaches are often not taken seriously and while they may be due to simple causes, they may also be symptoms of a deeper problem and just taking an aspirin may not be enough. The internationally renowned naturopath Dr Alfred Vogel explains it like this: 'When the church is on fire the bells are rung to warn people of the fire spreading. It is no use stopping the bells ringing, though it is easy enough to do so, that will not stop the fire. The only way to do that is to call the fire brigade.' Taking pain relievers for headaches may stop the pain. It will not cure the condition causing the pain.

Be it a simple headache or a severe migraine, never lose sight of the fact that the cause may be due to seemingly unrelated problems in the body or in the environment. While it is important to seek professional help, especially if the pain is severe, much can be achieved if you decide to take charge of your own health. However, it is no use going to any health care professional with the attitude, 'Cure me while I get on with my life as before'.

People perceive pain differently and have different pain thresholds, and there is still much to be learned about the mechanisms that transmit pain. Headaches are no exception, although it is known that anxiety and depression can make you more sensitive to them. A thorough understanding of the types of headaches and their possible causes will go a long way to prevent and eliminate many of the common headaches.

Headaches With Simple Causes

Weather

Cold, biting winds can cause the muscles of the head to contract and so cause pain. If the *frontalis muscle* is affected, the pain will be in the forehead. Similarly, *temporalis muscles* contraction will cause pain in the temples. Contraction of the *occipitalis muscles* will result in pain at the back of the head.

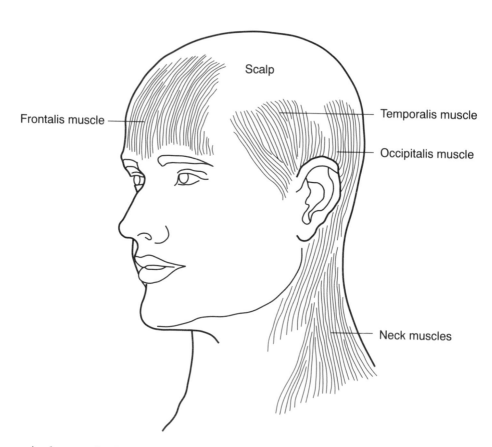

A change in *barometric* (atmospheric) pressure can sometimes cause headaches. So may dry winds.

Exercise Headaches

Strenuous exercise, particularly in hot weather or at high altitudes, can culminate in a throbbing headache. One explanation is that the brain has been starved of *glucose* (a form of sugar needed for energy) because it has been diverted to exercising muscles. It is said that in some people the blood vessels on the surface of the brain *dilate* (become wider or larger) during exercise and this may cause pain.

Altered Sleep – Too Much Or Too Little?

Sleeping for too long or, conversely, having too little sleep, can also cause headaches. Interrupted sleep may have the same effect.

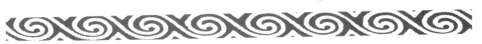

Fluorescent Lighting

Fluorescent lighting may be another cause of headaches.
Fluorescent lights which flicker at high frequency, and are therefore
not noticed, are the greatest culprits.

Travel

Setting off on a journey after too little sleep, anxiety about making a
plane connection, pressurised cabins, glare while driving in the sun,
and neck tension during long periods of driving are but a few of the
many factors which can contribute to headaches while travelling.

Food-Related Headaches

Many dietary factors cause headaches. These are discussed in detail
in Chapter 3.

Premenstrual Syndrome

Some women regularly have headaches before their periods are
due, starting from 2 to 7 days before menstruation. The most
popular explanation for this is that fluid retention (common in
women at this time) causes pressure on the brain.

Stuffy Atmospheres

Cigarette smoke, petrol fumes, paint and hair-spray can all trigger
headaches.

Sexual Headaches

Several types of headache are caused by sexual activity. A dull pain
may develop at the back of the head and becomes more
pronounced as sexual excitement increases. This is caused by the
contraction of the neck and head muscles. The sudden rise in blood
pressure that occurs during orgasm can also provoke headaches. In
some cases, headaches may become worse after sex (but on the
other hand, orgasms can alleviate certain types of headaches).

Cinema, TV And Reading

It is not uncommon for people to come out of the cinema with a

throbbing headache. In the same way, staring at a TV screen or a computer monitor, or prolonged reading, may bring one on. This may be due to continuous focusing on the screen or page.

Migraine

Some common headaches, together with other ailments of the twentieth century, can be attributed to the strains and stresses of Western civilisation. But the recorded history of migraine dates back to 80 AD when Aretaeus, a physician in Turkey, first defined what he called *heterocrania* – a pain affecting the right or left side of the head. A hundred years later the famous physician, Galen, gave the complaint the name *hermicrania*. The word 'migraine' is a corruption of that word, as was its first English derivative 'megrim'.

The rich, the powerful and the famous have all been victims of migraine. The list includes Julius Caeser, Edward Gibbon, John Calvin, Immanuel Kant, Friedrich Nietzsche, Thomas Jefferson, William Shakespeare, Alexander Pope, Lewis Carroll, Rudyard Kipling, George Elliot, Lewis Carroll and Sigmund Freud. But contrary to popular myth, migraine is not the exclusive privilege of the intelligent or powerful: migraine sufferers are to be found in every stratum of society. The picture of a 'migraine personality' as being perfectionist, very intelligent and hardworking may be due to the fact that a larger number of people in these categories seek medical advice. Most sufferers never consult a doctor.

While migraine may begin in childhood and continue into the 70s, it is a condition that mostly affects the younger generation. The average age of sufferers is around 38. Women are at least twice as likely to suffer than men, with the majority of women mostly affected in their reproductive years. Menstruation and oral contraceptives are known to contribute to the incidence of migraine. For some unknown reason, however, during pregnancy there are very few attacks, especially in the last six months. There is also a hereditary tendency, with migraine sufferers having a 60 per cent chance of having a relative with the ailment.

There have been many definitions of migraine since it was first recognised several hundred years ago. While committees of doctors have come up with long and complex definitions, one relatively simple, sensible description was supplied by a doctor called Valquist:

'a *paroxysmal* [sudden or uncontrollable] headache separated by headache-free intervals and accompanied by two of the following four features: *nausea* [feelings that precede vomiting], *focal cerebral symptoms* [vision disturbance], *unilaterality* [affecting one side of the head] and a positive family history'.

This clearly distinguishes it from tension and most other types of headaches, though they may have one or two features in common in certain individuals. The *Concise Oxford Dictionary* offers the following definition: 'recurrent throbbing headache that usually affects one side of the head, often accompanied by nausea and disturbance of vision'. A migraine can last anything from two hours to two days, and the sufferer may experience just a single attack, although recurrent attacks, at varying intervals, are more common.

Classic Migraine

This frequently runs in families and starts in childhood or adolescence. It tends to get better with age and in women is usually gone by the menopause .

A typical attack begins with the *aura* (visual disturbance, the sufferer sees haloes round objects, zig-zags, or flashing lights). Part of the field of vision may disappear on one side. More rarely, there may be a tingling sensation down one side of the body. The aura is followed by a headache, almost always on one side only, with nausea, vomiting and sensitivity to light, all of which last from 6 to 48 hours. In women, this sort of migraine is more common before a period. In pregnancy it may become more frequent, but 60 per cent of women are entirely headache-free at this time. Classic migraine may be brought on by the contraceptive pill. So women who suffer migraine should perhaps avoid this means of contraception.

Common Migraine

This is the commonest form of migraine and results in a one-sided or sometimes generalised headache. There is no aura and it tends to come on when a person is relaxing after a period of stress, typically at weekends only. It can be difficult to distinguish from a tension headache. Recent research has suggested that some sufferers have both types of headache and treatment should be given accordingly.

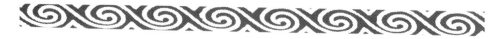

Cluster Headaches

One of the few migraine-types which is commoner in men, a succession of headaches occurs nightly for a period of 3 to 6 weeks and there may then be no further attacks for months or years. Alcohol may be a precipitating factor.

The pain is always unilateral over one eye. It builds to a crescendo, then lasts up to 2 hours and spreads, sometimes to the forehead, cheek and temple. The eye is often red and watery, the pupil may become smaller and the eyelid droop. These last two changes may persist for many hours after the headache. There may also be stuffiness in the nose and flushing of the face.

Vertebrobasilar Migraine

When the *vertebrobasilar vessels* (a group of blood vessels that supplies oxygen and nutrition to the neck and the *cerebellum* – the back of the brain, which is involved in balance and co-ordination) are affected by a migraine. There may be unsteadiness in walking, double vision and *vertigo* (dizziness). The pain is usually at the back of the head. These unpleasant symptoms are, thankfully, uncommon.

Facial Migraine

Pain is felt in the lower half of the face rather than in the temple area. The pain lasts longer than with cluster headaches and nausea and vomiting are more frequent.

Hemiplegic Migraine

A rare type of migraine, this is characterised by weakness of the limbs down one side of the body, which may last for several days even after the headache has gone. There is usually a family history but, if not, the person should be further investigated to exclude an abnormality of the blood vessels in the brain. If you do suffer weakness in the limbs, get a professional opinion.

Ophthalmoplegic Migraine

This migraine is round the eyes. The nerve supply to some of the muscles around the eyeball is temporarily interrupted so that there

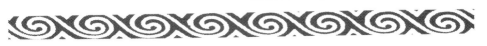

is the appearance of a squint and the eyes do not move in a co-ordinated way.

Status Migranosis

This rare condition is when the headache of a migraine continues unabated and vomiting is incessant. Dehydration may set in, so the person may need admission to hospital for intravenous fluids.

What Is The Cause Of Migraine?

Not only is there no agreement on the definition of 'migraine' but the cause is also a matter of debate.

Those in favour of the *vascular* theory say that when the blood vessels supplying the brain shut down (for reasons not yet known), the brain functions are affected as a result of the reduced blood supply, causing migraine. Other experts believe that in classic migraine, there is a reduction in the amount of blood flowing to the brain. When the minimum level of blood supply needed for the brain to function properly falls below a certain level, migraine symptoms manifest themselves.

The *neurological* theory suggests that migraine begins in the brain tissue and as a result the blood vessels shut down. It is like a person turning pale with fear – it is the emotion of fear that causes the constriction.

It can be said with some certainty that during a migraine attack there is an abnormality in the levels of *neurotransmitters* (the chemical messengers of the brain). Avoidance of foods containing these substances is helpful in reducing migraine attacks (see Chapter 3).

Platelets are cells that are responsible for repairing breaches in the lining of the blood vessels. It has been found that during a migraine attack there is a significant increase in the neurotransmitter *serotonin* that is released by the platelets. One of the main effects of serotonin is to constrict the blood vessels. Some authorities consider this to be the primary cause of migraine.

Food And Chemical Allergy Theory

There is a school of thought that believes that food allergy is perhaps the single most important cause of migraine and that all

others are secondary (see Chapter 3). There have been a number of trials all round the world which have concluded that food allergy accounts for 80 to 90 per cent of cases. What is surprising is that, in addition to the well-known triggers such as caffeine, common foods – wheat, corn, milk, cheese, chocolate and sugars – are all implicated in causing migraine.

Managing Headaches and Migraine

While the experts debate over the cause and cure of migraine, sufferers have no choice but to cope with this ailment. Often they have to stop whatever they are doing and retire to a darkened room to try to sleep and endure the debilitating pain.

While there is no 'cure' in terms of modern allopathic medicine, a thorough understanding of the triggers and the correct management of headaches and migraines can help avoid or, at least, to mitigate the symptoms.

The management of headaches and migraines has two elements: first, recognising the triggers and avoiding them and, second, what to do during an attack.

Chapter 2 describes what your GP can do for you. The third chapter highlights dietary considerations, and the subsequent chapters will describe the many complementary therapies available to you to help you to alleviate the pain and, more importantly, to prevent or ease the severity and frequency of attacks.

2

ORTHODOX MEDICINE: WHAT CAN YOUR GP OFFER?

Only 1 in 50 of us can say we never suffer from headaches. The rest of us, 98 per cent of the population, have to put up with them, trying to cope by ourselves by taking painkillers such as aspirin or paracetamol or just by resting quietly.

There are a number of unfortunate people who suffer from headaches frequently, or almost continuously, but are afraid to ask their doctor's opinion in case something serious is found. In fact, serious causes, such as brain tumours, are extremely rare and the average family doctor will come across a person with a brain tumour only once every 5 to 10 years. Any new, severe, or very persistent headache, however, is one you should take to your GP, as some conditions need urgent medical treatment.

Sorting out the cause of a headache can take a considerable time, and it is most important for your doctor to go into detail about the site, type and frequency of the pain.

Pains in the head may come from nearby structures, such as the *cervical spine* (bones in the neck), teeth, jaw or sinuses, as well as the ears, nose or throat. This type of pain is called *referred pain.*

It may be helpful to keep a diary of events – with activities, diet, alcohol intake, menstrual pattern and descriptions of the headaches – to establish whether there is a specific cause or trigger factor. This all takes a great deal of effort but is well worth the trouble if the right treatment can be found.

Quite often there is a simple explanation and a change of habit is all that is needed. Not every pain in the head needs a prescription! *Clinical investigations* (investigations based on observation) of headaches are not usually necessary but your doctor may request them if the cause cannot easily be found or if the pain is not responding as expected. Alternatively, a specialist, usually a *neurologist* (a doctor who specialises in diseases of the nervous system), may see you and request tests.

Common tests are skull X-rays, looking at the bones both inside and outside of the skull, and *CT scans* (where serial pictures of 'slices' of the brain are taken). This can give a great deal of information about the brain itself. *Arteriography* may be needed. This is where dye is injected into a main blood vessel in the neck and X-rays are taken to show details of circulation in the brain. *Lumbar puncture*, where a small needle is inserted into the lower end of the *spinal canal* (duct of the spine), in the *lumbar region* (the part of the body between the lower ribs and the hips) is sometimes helpful. Samples of fluid are extracted and tested for a variety of substances. This test is essential if *meningitis* (inflammation of the membranes that surround the brain and spinal cord) is suspected.

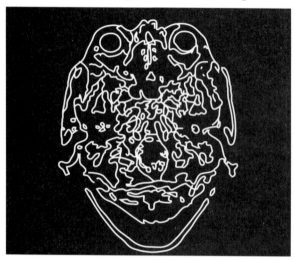

In this CT scan of a human head, the cross-section of the eyeballs can be seen at the top of the photograph.

By far the commonest types of headache are migraine and tension headaches and treatment for these will be dealt with in some detail. Both of these may be brought on by stress. It is easy to recommend changes in lifestyle to reduce anxiety but practical advice on what to change and how this should be done is not always forthcoming from the family doctor. Among GPs generally, there seems to be an increasing acceptance of complementary therapies for the treatment of headaches. Many people, once they know that the cause of their problem is not life threatening, prefer to try alternative therapies rather than resort to prescription medicines. Yoga, meditation and hypnosis are being recommended more frequently, as are aromatherapy and other treatments (see later chapters).

Tension Headaches

The pain of a tension headache is characteristically dull, constant and *slowly progressive* (advancing slowly by steps or degrees). It occurs at the back of the head and neck or as a band-like pain all the way round and is probably related as much to muscular tension as emotional tension. There is no vomiting. The patient coming in to see his/her GP may have had continuous pain for weeks or months and this sort of history alone almost excludes any other cause. Apart from some tenderness at the back of the neck, examination reveals that everything else is completely normal.

Treatment

Tension headaches are notoriously resistant to the usual painkillers. This is why many people visit their doctor, believing that there must be something very seriously wrong. It is often difficult to reassure a sufferer who is expecting a prescription that the real, long-term answer is a change of habits and paying more attention to relaxation and lifestyle.

While it is easy to prescribe very strong painkillers, such as *dihydrocodeine,* or one of the many *anti-inflammatory drugs* (drugs that reduce swelling), such as *naproxen* (trade name: Naprosyn) or *ibuprofen* (trade name: Nurofen), even these are unlikely to affect the pain. Some other treatments do seem to work, however, and recent studies have suggested that treatments used for migraine can be effective in tension headaches. These are described briefly below.

Antidepressants

People are often confused about the differences between these drugs and *tranquillisers* (drugs that calm a person) but, in fact, antidepressants act on the brain in a completely different way from tranquillisers and do not have the same potential for addiction. Antidepressants are effective in raising the pain threshold, although the sufferer may not complain of symptoms of depression. They are used for a variety of conditions where chronic pain is a feature. It is not entirely clear why they work but they are one of the most effective *nonanalgesic* (a substance that does not work by producing an inability to feel pain) treatments for reducing pain.

There is a wide variety of tablets available, some of which are relatively sedative, for example, *prothiaden* (trade name: Dothiepin),

amitriptylline (trade name: Tryptizol). These are helpful if sleep is disturbed. Others have little effect on alertness, for example, *fluoxetine* (trade name: Prozac), and are taken in the morning. As with most other treatments for tension headaches, their effect is not felt immediately. For most people 10 to 14 days' treatment is necessary before there is any improvement. A course will last for at least 6 to 8 weeks, often months, and the tablets are then tailed off gradually over a couple of weeks. They should never be stopped suddenly because of the risk of withdrawal effects, which could include irregular heartbeat. Although care is needed when mixing tablets, they may be taken with most over-the-counter painkillers. It is best to ask your doctor's advice first.

Beta Blockers

These are useful as an interim measure, especially for anxious patients. They are generally given as a course over a few weeks, occasionally months, until the headache subsides or until a more suitable treatment can be found. Their particular advantage is that they are not potentially addictive. Many people find this reassuring and are more willing to take them than, say, antidepressants.

Sumatriptan

A recent trial using the drug *sumatriptan* to treat patients with tension headache showed that it had a small but significant effect. It is unlikely, though, that it will become a standard treatment as it is an expensive drug and does not encourage people to consider the necessary changes in lifestyle that would make their headaches less frequent.

Tranquillisers

These, for example, *diazepam* (trade name: Valium) and *lorazepam* (trade name: Ativan) may seem the obvious answer for someone who is tense and anxious, especially since they also help to relax the muscles. In fact, they are rarely prescribed for tension headaches because of their great potential for addiction. It is well known that a high proportion of tension-headache sufferers overuse painkillers and experience withdrawal symptoms from them as well as increased headaches. Tranquillisers are therefore best reserved for acute anxiety alone and, even then, in short courses supervised by the GP.

Headaches Which Need Urgent Treatment

Certain serious conditions may start as a headache. Immediate treatment is important and could be life saving. In general, whenever a headache comes on suddenly, is not responsive to ordinary painkillers or is accompanied by a rash, drowsiness or vomiting, the advice of a doctor should be sought at once.

Temporal Arteritis

This condition occurs almost exclusively in people over the age of 55. It frequently produces a severe headache on one side, mainly around the temple, with tenderness of this area. It is diagnosed by taking a sample of the blood vessel from the temple under local anaesthetic and examining it for inflammation. A blood test called the *erythrocyte sedimentation rate (ESR)* can help to measure the inflammation as well. The main artery to the eye may be affected and this can lead to blindness if not treated promptly.

The treatment is with oral steroids, usually *prednisolone* tablets (trade name: Prednisone), which are given in high doses initially and then gradually reduced. While steroids have many possible side-effects, there is no other suitable orthodox treatment and under medical supervision most people remain well while taking them. Steroids may need to be continued for months, or even years, and progress is monitored with ESR blood tests at regular intervals.

Hypertension

The majority of people with *hypertension* (high blood pressure) do not get headaches unless the blood pressure level is extremely high. However, in rare cases, the pressure may rise rapidly causing a headache which is severe and unresponsive to normal painkillers and is called *malignant hypertension.* Urgent hospital treatment is needed and drugs are often given through a drip to bring the condition under control quickly. Tablet treatment is then continued for life, as in most cases of hypertension.

The same sort of problem may occur as a temporary illness during pregnancy. This is called *pre-eclampsia.* For reasons that are still unknown, there is a sudden onset of symptoms including headache and swelling of the ankles. There is nearly always protein found in the urine. There is also a rise in blood pressure, although this may

be much less than in severe hypertension, and hospital admission is necessary. The baby may sometimes need to be delivered early if drug treatment with tablets or by drip cannot control the blood pressure. If the blood pressure is very high an *eclamptic fit* (convulsion) may occur, but this is uncommon. Once the baby is born, the symptoms usually subside rapidly. Recent trials have shown that low doses of aspirin can be helpful in preventing eclampsia and many previous sufferers are now given this drug throughout subsequent pregnancies.

Glaucoma

Mostly a disease of the middle-aged and the elderly, *glaucoma* involves raised pressure within the eyeball. In its chronic form, the pressure usually rises slowly with a gradual loss of vision. Then a headache over and around the eye may develop. Acute glaucoma, however, comes on suddenly and is often accompanied by flashing lights in the field of vision. The eye becomes red and the pain around the eye and over the forehead is severe and constant in nature. Vision becomes markedly reduced. Prompt medical treatment is needed to safeguard the sight in that and the other eye. Sometimes an injection of a drug called *diazoxide* is needed to reduce the pressure rapidly. An emergency operation is sometimes performed to release the pressure of fluid in one of the chambers of the eye. Many people control the pressure with regular insertion of eyedrops, for example, *timolol* (trade name: Timoptol) or *pilocarpine.* Pilocarpine, however, has the effect of constricting the pupil and may reduce the ability of the eye to focus.

Tumours

The diagnosis of a brain tumour is one which many people fear, if their headaches are prolonged or severe. The vast majority of people will be reassured by a visit to their GP that this is not the case. However, a progressively worsening headache with blackouts or vomiting should always be taken seriously. In fact, only a third of people with a tumour go to their doctor with a headache. Symptoms of a tumour are more usually personality change, an epileptic fit, or persistent disturbance of vision, all of which need investigation by a specialist as soon as possible.

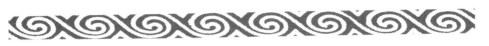

Meningitis

This potentially life-threatening illness occurs when the protective membrane around the brain becomes inflamed due to a virus or bacterium.

There has been increased media coverage of this illness recently, mainly because the disease can be difficult to diagnose in young children. Although, in all probability, many children develop a headache, they are unable to describe it and so the only visible signs of illness will be a reluctance to feed, vomiting and a temperature. In one of the most serious forms, *meningococcal meningitis*, a red, blotchy rash appears and at this stage very urgent antibiotic treatment is needed, with admission to hospital. Older children and adults usually develop a headache with vomiting and drowsiness. The neck becomes stiff and the eyes sensitive to bright light.

The only way to tell which sort of meningitis is present is for the person to undergo a lumbar puncture in hospital. A sample of fluid is immediately examined under a microscope and *cultured* (grown in a nutrient substance) to see which bacteria or viruses grow. *Bacterial meningitis* is always treated with antibiotics in high doses through a drip. *Viral meningitis* usually just resolves by itself, although the patient needs to be monitored and given painkillers until recovery.

A vaccine against one of the more serious infections, *haemophilus meningitis*, is now being given routinely to children and this offers protection against this form of the illness.

Subarachnoid Haemorrhage

Here there is leaking of blood from the vessels around the brain. It may occur in people of any age but is more usual over the age of 40. Sometimes there is a dilation of part of a vessel, called an *aneurysm*, which ruptures. It can also happen as the result of an injury to the brain and a number of other causes.

In most cases, the headache is sudden and severe, and is often described as 'like being hit over the head with a blunt instrument'. Neck stiffness is prominent, followed by loss of consciousness. The person needs to be admitted to hospital immediately. It is sometimes necessary to repair or tie off the vessel by an operation, but if the bleeding is minor it may stop without any treatment. High blood pressure will predispose a person to this condition.

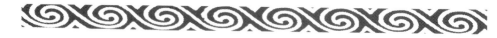

Depression

Particularly in people over the age of 45, a headache may be the first and only sign of depression, which can be very serious in some cases. Other features maybe lack of energy, disturbed sleep and low mood, loss of libido, and feelings of guilt and unworthiness. A change in personality is important and should always be promptly investigated to exclude the possibility of a brain tumour. It is impossible to generalise about treatment, as it varies from individual to individual.

Common Causes Of Headaches

Sinusitis

This condition often gives rise to headaches and facial pain. The sinuses are cavities within the bones of the face, lying behind the nose, in the centre of the forehead and within the cheekbones. Each sinus is lined with a membrane which secretes mucus and each is connected to the main nasal passage by small holes. When the holes become blocked for any reason, mucus collects and is unable to escape. Sinusitis may be *chronic* (of long duration) or *acute* (of short duration), causing generalised illness and sometimes obvious swelling of the face.

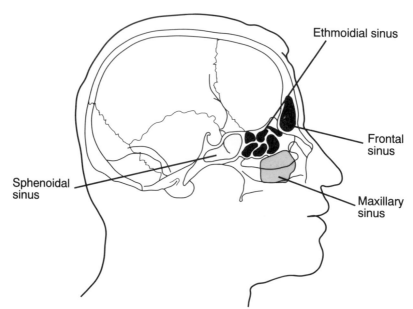

Paranasal sinuses seen in median view

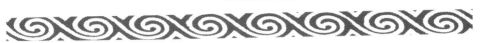

Treatment

Almost every sufferer is likely to benefit from inhalation of steam, with or without the addition of another preparation, such as eucalyptus, and this, combined with *analgesics* (painkillers) available over the counter, is sufficient for most people. A very acute episode, though, with a temperature or a lot of pain, will need antibiotics, for example, *amoxycillin* or *cephalexin* (trade names: Amoxil, Keflex), and stronger analgesics from the doctor.

Decongestant sprays are available over the counter as well as on prescription. These can give temporary relief but their effects tend to wear off quickly and they are probably no more effective than steam alone. Nasal drops, such as *ephedrine*, also do this but there can be a 'rebound' effect, that is, worsening of the symptoms when they are stopped, so they should only be used for a day or two.

Chronic sufferers may have a miserable time, with persistent headaches and blocked nose. Quite often an injury to the nose will result in deformity of the *nasal septum* (the piece of cartilage dividing the nose in the midline) and this can make the condition worse. The only answer here is surgical correction of the deformity, with opening and draining of the sinuses.

Dental Pain

It is surprising how often teeth, especially *impacted* (unable to come through) wisdom teeth, can cause pain which is felt as a headache. It is always worth checking with your dentist, if you are in your teens or twenties, to see if they are the cause of the problem. Whatever your age, a check-up is worthwhile to exclude a tooth abscess.

Drugs

There is a long list of prescribed medicines and tablets which can cause headaches. These include drugs used for heart disease and hypertension, for example, *bendrofluazide* and other *diuretics* (drugs that increase the flow of urine), such as *nifedipine* (trade name: Adalat) and *glyceryl trinitrate*. Even *atenolol* and other B blockers, which are used effectively in migraine, can cause headaches in a minority of people.

Antidepressants may also cause headaches. The two main types used are *tricyclics*, for example, *amitriptylline*, and *monoamine oxidase inhibitors*, for example, Nardil (trade name). There are dietary restrictions with the latter drug and certain foods may cause a

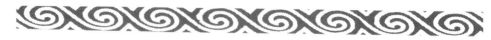

dangerous rise in blood pressure if taken with the drug. Your doctor will give you a list of these foods if you are prescribed this type of medication. Whatever the tablet, if you develop a headache after taking it, see your doctor straightaway.

Other Causes Of Headache

Trigeminal Neuralgia

The *trigeminal nerve* supplies sensation to the face and the eye and has three main branches, one for each part of the face. For reasons that are unclear, the nerve becomes irritated and causes a severe, usually stabbing, pain on one side of the face and scalp. There may be a few weeks of this recurrent pain, which subsides only to return at a later date. Treatment is generally with *carbamazepine* tablets. This drug reduces the abnormal nerve impulses to the face (and is also used for epilepsy, where it stops the nerve impulses which cause convulsions). The dose is built up gradually to avoid side-effects. Most people tolerate it fairly well but it can itself cause headaches and a variety of symptoms, including unsteady gait and a rash. Levels of the drug need to be monitored from time to time with blood tests.

Post-herpetic Neuralgia (Shingles)

Shingles is caused by the virus *herpes zoster* and may affect the trigeminal nerve, as above. The pain is generally constant and may precede the typical blistery rash. Treatment is the same as for trigeminal neuralgia if standard painkillers do not work, that is, gradually increasing doses of *carbamazepine*. Both types of neuralgia may be treated with antidepressants.

Post-traumatic Headache

When a person sustains a head injury the brain is shaken up inside the skull. If there is loss of consciousness, then the person is said to have concussion. Luckily, lasting damage is rare, even if there is a fracture of the skull, but post-concussion headache is common. It is now accepted that it is mostly a tension-type headache rather than a direct result of the injury. Treatment is with the usual simple painkillers. The headache may last for months after the injury.

Cervical Spondylosis

The vertebrae in the neck can become squashed together by wear-and-tear, injury or *arthritis* (inflammation of the joints). When this

happens the nerves emerging between the vertebrae in the neck become squashed and cause pain which can radiate to the scalp.

Treatment is with physiotherapy, sometimes with manipulation of the bones. Anti-inflammatory painkillers are helpful for some, for example, *ibuprofen* (trade name: Neurofen) and *fenbufen*. A surgical collar can be beneficial if pain is severe, but this is discouraged for long-term use as it tends to make the neck muscles weak and people may become very reliant upon it.

Migraine

As was made clear in the last chapter, despite many years of research, there is no clear agreement among orthodox medical practitioners as to the true cause of migraine. One of two current theories revolves around an abnormality of blood vessels in and around the brain. These blood vessels contract in response to certain chemicals, and this causes visual disturbance. Then those arteries around the brain expand and this causes pain. The second theory is that the abnormality starts within the brain itself with a kind of partial 'shutting down' and following this the arteries expand and contract in response.

So far, no cure has been found for migraine and even the latest and best treatment is thought to be only 60 per cent effective. The most important part of treatment is understanding what makes migraine come on, what trigger factors exist and what can be done to avoid them.

Foods are well-known trigger factors, although many sufferers will say from experience that food and other triggers do not reliably cause migraine and that there is often a threshold of a certain amount of a food which has to be reached before the trigger will 'work'. Coffee, oranges, red wine and other forms of alcohol, cheese and chocolate are all common triggers. Tension, pregnancy, sleep deprivation and many other factors can also be responsible. It is not unusual for no trigger at all to be found.

It has been said by some doctors that the term 'migraine' is used far too often to describe all sorts of headaches in order to make them more acceptable to other people. 'Having a migraine' probably does generate more sympathy than, say, having a tension headache, which always implies that the person concerned is weak or can't cope. It is essential, though, for the family doctor to take a full history of the type of headache and to try and be absolutely sure

there is no other cause. There are many different types of migraine and each has a specific treatment. Most people, however, have either classic or common migraine as described in Chapter 1.

Referral to a specialist is not often necessary. A *neurologist*, a consultant in diseases of the nervous system, may be able to help with treatment and, if the diagnosis is not clear, may arrange some of the investigations described earlier. There are a few centres, such as The Migraine Clinic in London, which offer very specialised advice and treatment for persistent and debilitating headache symptoms.

Migraine Treatment

General Measures During An Attack

It is very important to use common sense and to stop working during an attack. Lying down in a darkened room and sleeping may abort an attack, or at least shorten it, if carried out soon enough. Pressure on the part of the head that is painful, in conjunction with local heat, perhaps provided by a hot water bottle, is sometimes helpful, too. Simple analgesics, such as paracetamol and aspirin, are often sufficient to control the pain. All medicines should be taken with a drink and as early in the attack as possible. Migraine slows down the emptying of the stomach and will delay the absorption of tablets if they are taken later.

Anti-emetics

This group of drugs is essential for those who find vomiting and retching as much of a problem as the pain of migraine.

Metoclopramide (trade name: Maxolon) is useful as it helps the stomach to empty, something which can be greatly delayed during an attack. It can be given orally, by injection into the muscle or, more rarely, by intravenous injection.

Prochlorperazine (trade name: Stemetil) is also a useful drug and may be given in tablet or suppository form. *Cyclizine* is another such drug. Some products combine a painkiller with an anti-emetic, for example, Migraleve (trade name), which contains paracetamol, codeine and the anti-emetic *buclizine* and is available over the counter.

All anti-emetics may cause drowsiness, desirable for those people who are resting at the time of an attack, but care is needed when, for example, driving and operating machinery. The recommended dose should never be exceeded.

Sumatriptan (Trade Name: Imigran)

This drug can only be used for an acute attack and not for prevention. One of the newest drugs for migraine, *sumatriptan,* acts by blocking the action of one of the body's chemical transmitters, *5 hydroxy-tryptamine,* which acts on the brain, at nerve endings and on blood vessels. Initially, it was brought out only in injectable form to be given deep under the skin but it is now also available as tablets. The first injection is usually given by a doctor but the injection kit is designed for patients to use themselves once they have been properly taught how to do this.

The speed of action can be remarkable in some people, with a full recovery in less than half an hour. One repeat dose only may be given within a 24-hour period. It may cause drowsiness in some individuals. Since it can cause spasm in the arteries, it is to be used with caution by people with heart disease and high blood pressure.

With such a treatment available it is, of course, tempting not to address the important issues, which concern lifestyle and trigger factors. As long as this temptation is avoided, it is a very useful drug for those people who have occasional, very debilitating episodes of migraine.

Preventive Treatments

Pizotifen (Trade Name: Sanomigran)

Pizotifen comes in tablet and liquid form. It acts by blocking the action of one of the chemicals in the brain which transmits the sensation of pain. This substance is called *serotonin.*

Pizotifen is usually given at night as it may cause drowsiness. Other possible side-effects are weight-gain, nausea, dizziness, muscle pains and mood changes. The dose is increased gradually over 2 or 3 weeks and is continued for several weeks, often as a trial, as it does not work for everybody. It is useful to keep a diary before and during the treatment period to assess any change in the pattern of headaches.

Beta Blockers

These drugs, for example, *atenolol* (trade name: Tenormin) and *propranolol* (trade name: Inderal), are used for a variety of conditions, including high blood pressure and angina. They may also be effective for anxiety and tension headaches. They act on the circulatory system, mainly to prevent the effects of fear and of exertion on the body, that is, they damp down the 'fight or flight' mechanism that is usually triggered by adrenaline, slowing the pulse rate and reducing blood pressure.

The exact way in which they prevent migraine is not very clear but it is probably connected to their ability to stabilise blood vessels in and around the brain, stopping them from expanding and contracting. They also have the effect of slightly constricting the airways to the lungs. This does not affect most people but can cause asthmatics to wheeze more and become short of breath, so they need to be used with caution.

Beta blockers are given in tablet form, although liquid is available. They can cause a variety of side-effects including nausea, vomiting, diarrhoea and insomnia but these are generally well tolerated in most people. Lassitude and ataxia may occur. Sensory sensations in the hands, blood disorders, skin rashes and hallucinations may occur, but less frequently. Heart failure and wheezing may also occur. A change to a slightly different formula can sometimes help. They must not be given with *ergotamine.*

Ergotamine

One of the first preventive treatments for migraine, it is still a useful drug for those people who have severe attacks. It acts by constricting the arteries in the brain. It has no effect on the *aura* (visual disturbance) of a classic migraine and can make vomiting worse, so is often given with an anti-emetic. Two types of tablets are available, one to be swallowed, for example, Cafergot (trade name), the other to be dissolved under the tongue, for example, Lingraine (trade name). A nasal spray is also available which some people find more convenient to use. An injectable form exists but is seldom used as sumatriptan is safer and in most cases just as effective.

At one time ergotamine was the only really effective treatment for severe migraine and some sufferers tended to overuse it. This resulted in headaches as a side-effect of treatment, so it is important that the maximum dose is not exceeded in any day or week. Suddenly stopping the tablets can provoke headaches, too, so this

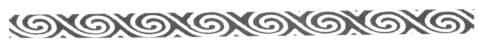

should always be done under the supervision of a doctor.

Abdominal pain can occur as a side-effect of ergotamine. Chronic overuse can also, very rarely, cause circulatory problems in the legs from prolonged arterial constriction, and gangrene may develop. Ergotamine interacts with several other drugs and your doctor will advise you as to what you are allowed to take with it.

Methysergide
This drug is not used very often but can be helpful for some of the less common migraine variants, such as cluster headaches, migranous neuralgia and severe migraine associated with menstruation. It is given in tablet form. Like ergotamine it has a constricting effect on blood vessels and should only be used under medical supervision, with a review every few weeks.

Anyone with circulation problems should not use it. Side-effects include drowsiness, nausea and disturbance of sleep. A rare side-effect is *fibrosis* (thickening of tissue) of the lungs and *pericardium* (the covering of the heart). Despite its potential hazards, however, it may be the only effective drug for some people.

Antidepressants
These are useful for a few patients for reasons that are not clearly understood.

Clonidine (Trade Name: Dixarit)
This drug has been around for many years and is occasionally used to control menopausal flushes. Today, it is seldom used for migraine but is worth trying if other tablets fail. It may have a stabilising effect on blood vessels but its mode of action is unclear. The dose is gradually built up over 2 or 3 weeks. Side-effects include dry mouth, drowsiness and constipation. Slowing of the heart rate may occur in the first few weeks of treatment. It may produce impotence, itching, swelling of the throat and face, nausea, and dizziness.

Carbimazepine And Phenytoin
Both these drugs are used occasionally. They have a stabilising effect on brain activity and are used commonly for epilepsy. It is unlikely they would be prescribed other than by a specialist.

Steroids
Short courses of oral steroids, for example, *prednisolone*, can be helpful for cluster headaches and in *status migranosis* (recurrent migraines) if other treatments fail.

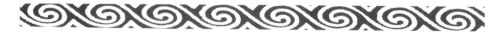

Conclusion

It should be clear that your GP has a wide range of drugs which may help you, at his or her disposal – but never let the success of a drug in alleviating your pain make you forget about investigating the underlying cause or trigger.

3

NUTRITION: THE PROBLEM LIES IN YOUR FOOD, NOT YOUR HEAD

As has already been mentioned, food and common headaches are interconnected. Fasting, or even a missed meal, bring on the pangs of hunger and, more often than not, a headache. As soon as you have some food inside you the sinking feeling disappears, as does the headache – unless you leave it so late to eat that the pain has developed into a full, throbbing headache. This is just a simple illustration of the strong link between food and headaches. But there is, in fact, much more to it than that. For example, a number of food substances trigger common headaches and simply avoiding the triggers will eliminate the headaches.

Common Triggers

Some common triggers of headaches and migraine

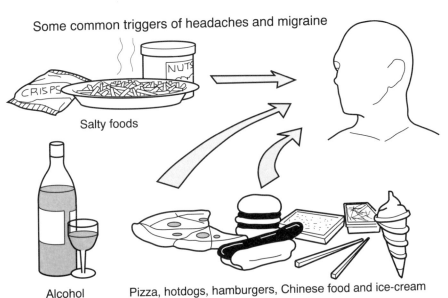

Salty foods

Alcohol

Pizza, hotdogs, hamburgers, Chinese food and ice-cream

Hunger Headaches

When you go for a long time without food your blood-sugar level drops and one symptom is a headache. So start your day with a good breakfast and, if you can, eat several small meals during the day. Snacks made from high-protein foods, such as beans, peas, nuts, seeds and lean meat, or wholegrain snacks may help. However, eating light snacks, especially those made from processed foods, instead of proper meals will aggravate the problem.

Salt Headaches

There is nothing inherently wrong with salt itself. It is the amount we consume that causes concern. On average we eat 8 to 12 g salt a day whereas we only really need 3 to 5 g. Some salt is naturally present in the foods we eat and some comes from what we add. However, most of our salt intake can be attributed to processed foods where salt has been added as a preservative to prevent foods going bad. Heavily salted snacks, such as crisps, chips and nuts, especially on an empty stomach, cause a sudden salt overload. Eliminating excessive salt from your everyday diet will help to reduce headaches.

Caffeine Withdrawal Headaches

If you are a caffeine addict, drinking 10 to 30 cups of tea or coffee, or even more, a day, and suddenly decide to kick the habit, you may develop headaches which last for up to 6 hours. Caffeine is known to constrict the blood vessels and its sudden withdrawal causes the blood vessels to dilate, giving you a headache. Try and reduce your caffeine addiction gradually. (For further details on caffeine addiction see *Alcohol, Smoking, Tranquillisers* in the Headway Healthwise series.)

Hot Dog Headache

Chemicals called *nitrites* and *nitrates* are added as preservatives to sausages and other meats to keep them looking fresh. These chemicals dilate the blood vessels in the head and may bring on headaches. Avoid all types of processed meats if you think these preservatives are the culprits.

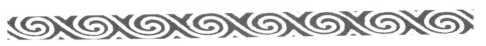

Chinese Food Headache

Monosodium glutamate (MSG), a chemical used as a flavour enhancer in soya sauce and many other foods, is the main cause of headaches that occur after eating Chinese food in a restaurant. A long wait for the food to be served may create the conditions for a hunger headache which, in turn, add to the likelihood of a headache after the meal. A few progressive restaurants in the USA now advertise their food as 'MSG free'. MSG is also used in canned foods and in some bottled sauces. Check food labels if you suspect that you are sensitive to MSG (check 'E' numbers).

Pizza Headache

Cheese can cause headaches as well. It contains *tyramine,* a by-product of the fermentation process. Yellow cheese has more tyramine than white cheese. Avoid, or at least limit, cheese intake. Be brave and ask for pizza without the cheese. Tyramine is also found in chicken and beef livers, as well as sour cream, salami, meat tenderisers and chocolate.

Ice-cream Headaches

Ice-cold foods and drinks can cause headaches. This is because the sudden cooling in the mouth activates the nerves which bring on the headache. It is said that cold makes the muscles of the palate and nose tighten up, resulting in a painful spasm. Eat slowly and only a little at a time.

Alcohol Headaches

This variety is not just restricted to the 'morning after' hangover! Drinking on an empty stomach can also cause a headache. Essentially, alcohol is a *vasodilater* (it dilates the blood vessels). This is further exacerbated by the additives which give a drink its individual taste.

There is no dearth of explanations, and suggestions, for hangover headaches. For example, it is thought that alcohol dehydrates the body. Drinking a pint of water before retiring is said to help. Alcohol can also upset blood glucose levels. However, the only sure way of eliminating alcohol-related headaches is simply not to drink alcohol at all!

Understanding Food Allergies And Intolerances

It is obvious that avoiding the foods which trigger the types of headaches described on the previous pages will have the desired effect. But what if the headaches and migraines are the result of food allergies? It is here that we enter into the realms of controversy. Before we can even discuss diet, we must look at the whole question of food allergies and intolerance.

A food allergy is an *inappropriate immunological response* (a reaction by the body to foreign materials) to foods or food ingredients normally tolerated by most people. There are two types of food allergies, *fixed* and *variable*. A person with a *fixed* allergic response reacts to even a small amount of a food every time it is encountered. The response is usually immediate.These people never seem to outgrow their allergies.

The more common type of allergic response is the *variable* response. This is more difficult to identify. It depends on the 'dose' and does not necessarily produce the same response, or even one at all, every time. More often than not, the response is delayed. It is therefore all the more difficult to diagnose. Just to add to the confusion, there is also disagreement among medical practitioners, and even among nutritionists, on the very definition of the term. Some insist that real allergies are quite rare compared to the more common food intolerances which can be associated with poor digestion, micronutrient-poor food and a weakened immune system.

An abnormal physiological response to food, which cannot be proven to be an immunological response (a reaction to foreign bodies) is generally referred to as *food intolerance.*

Migraine and Food

Food allergy or intolerance is perhaps the major cause of migraines. A number of recent carefully controlled trials have shown that identification and removal of the offending food can reduce or eliminate the symptoms of migraine in most sufferers.

However, the food – migraine connection is not a new finding. In 1873, a Dr Liveing published an account of migraines called *On megrim, Sick Headaches and some Allied Disorders*, in which he records wine and burnt pastry as causes. In this century, it was Dr Albert Rowe who first reported that, of the 48 patients with migraine in his

trials, almost all found complete relief after they had followed elimination diets. Indeed, the elimination diet is an important diagnostic tool for exposing food allergies (see 'Elimination Diet' page 48). Following Dr Rowe's work, many studies were undertaken in the USA. The results of the first British trials were published in May 1979 in the medical journal, the *Lancet*. Dr Ellen Grant of the Charing Cross Hospital, London, reported that 85 per cent of the 60 patients in her food allergy study became migraine free after the allergy had been identified. Another study on 88 children with migraine was reported in the *Lancet* in October 1983. Ninety-three per cent had significant improvement of their symptoms by following a low-risk allergy diet. The foods causing migraine were identified by introducing the foods one by one following an elimination diet.

How foods induce migraines is not clear. We have known for many years that red wine, chocolate and cheese, which all contain tyramine, can trigger a migraine. Tyramine, together with other substances such as serotonin, tryptamine and dopamine, has the effect of constricting the blood vessels. Migraine sufferers, it is thought, are deficient in an enzyme called *monoamine oxidase* which normally metabolises such substances, thus reducing their constricting effects.

Foods Which Are Commonly Thought To Induce Migraine

Cow's milk	Onions	Corn
Wheat	Soy	Oats
Chocolate	Pork	Cane sugar
Eggs	Peanuts	Yeast
Oranges	Alcohol	Apples
Benzoic acid	Monosodium	Peaches
Cheese	glutamate	Potatoes
Tomatoes	Walnuts	Chicken
Tartrazine	Beef	Bananas
Rye	Tea	Strawberries
Rice	Coffee	Melons
Fish	Nuts	Carrots
Grapes	Goats milk	

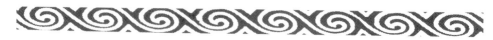

Hidden Allergy

Tracking down the particular food that causes a migraine may be more complicated than it first appears, as there may be a *hidden allergy*. This was first described by a well-known allergist, Dr Herbert Rinkel. A hidden allergy (or masked allergy) is one that causes the symptoms but the patient is unable to determine which substance causes the allergy.

It is easy to identify a food as the culprit when you come out in a rash or suffer a migraine attack every time it is consumed. However, if you are allergic to a food that is eaten daily or at least several times a week, it becomes very difficult to identify it, because the body becomes accustomed to the food and the reaction is dampened.

Dr Rinkel himself developed *allergic rhinitis*, a condition similar to hay fever with persistent nasal discharge. When all the normal tests failed to detect an allergen it made him focus on food. It so happened that during his medical studies his principal diet had been eggs. His father was an egg merchant and had been sending him vast quantities of eggs as a way of supporting him as a student. This high intake of eggs continued even after Dr Rinkel qualified. One day he consumed a rather large quantity of eggs to provoke a reaction. Instead, his allergic rhinitis actually improved a little. After a while he abstained from eggs completely. To his surprise there was a significant improvement in nasal symptoms. Five days later he happened to eat a piece of angel cake. He collapsed and his allergic rhinitis returned with a vengeance. An acute observer, Rinkel tried to replicate this by reintroducing his egg consumption and then omitting it for five days and then eating an egg again. Just as he had suspected, he collapsed and his nasal discharge returned. A number of experiments followed which supported his observations. Masked allergy has now gained currency among many medical practitioners.

In his book, *The Migraine Revolution* (Thorsons), Dr John Mansfield, one of the pioneers of allergy research in this country, writes:

'The concept of masking is the single most important fact to grasp about migraine. It explains the sorts of observations about migraine which have long been mysterious. It explains for a start why people prone to migraine who fast almost invariably get a migraine – because they are missing their next dose of their allergen. Hence it shows why migraine is so common amongst Jewish people on the Day of Atonement. Secondly, it explains why migraine specialists have found from experience that their patients will get less migraine if they have small frequent meals. They therefore advise them to eat very regularly. It

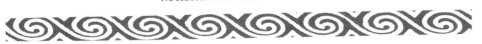

furthermore reveals why the commonest time to acquire a migraine is on awakening, because at this time of the day it has been many hours since the migraine sufferer consumed his last dose of allergic food, particularly if it was not present in his evening meal. It explains why many patients have a migraine on a Saturday. On this day they tend to lie in bed for longer than during the week and have breakfast later and therefore there is some delay in the time before they have their next masking feeding.'

This broadens the number of possible allergens to include milk, wheat, corn, eggs, etc., all of which are part of our daily diet and where the allergy can only be identified by the withdrawal response. Practitioners recommend a *rotation diet* to enable identification of the allergen. Please refer to the glossary on page 117, for an explanation of the procedure.

Chemical Allergy

There is an interesting story about one of the patients of Dr Randolph of Chicago. This patient used to get headaches whenever he ate apples. He then discovered that whenever he ate apples from a particular old orchard he did not get a headache. Upon further investigation it was discovered that this orchard had not been sprayed for some time. Dr Randolph tested this further by feeding him with several apples. Some of them had been sprayed and some not. Consistently, the patient only responded with a headache to the sprayed ones. It was obvious that the patient was not reacting to the fruit but to the residue of the spray.

Apples are often coated with paraffin wax to improve their shelf life, as well as appearance. Green bananas are ripened artificially by exposing them to ethylene gas. Corn is soaked in sulphur dioxide solution to stop fermentation. Additives in our foods, cigarette smoke, plastics, foams and aerosols can all contribute to an allergic response resulting in the symptoms of a migraine. An elimination diet can help to identify any offending food substance, if it is diet-related.

Nutritional Supplements

Most health food shops, and some pharmacists, stock a wide range of dietary supplements and some of them can be very useful indeed for people who suffer from migraines and headaches.

Fish Oil

Reducing the consumption of animal fats and increasing the consumption of fish oils has been known to help migraine victims. At the University of Cincinnati College of Medicine, eight patients with severe migraine received vegetable oil capsules with meals for 6 weeks followed by a substitution of fish oil capsules for 6 weeks. The fish oil capsules cut the incidence of severe headaches by more than half. In another study, reported in the *American Journal of Clinical Nutrition*, of six patients given 20 g fish oil daily, five found significant relief.

Quercetin

Quercetin, helpful in mitigating the effects of inflammation in allergies, has a molecular structure very similar to *sodium cromoglycate*, a drug that gives protection from foods known to induce attacks and may itself give protection.

Niacin

This water-soluble B vitamin has long been known for its vasodilatory effects and has been used in the treatment of migraine.

Magnesium

Beneficial in relaxing muscles.

Supplementation Programme

Quercetin – 500 mg per day   Niacin – 50 mg per day
Fish oils – 2 g per day   Magnesium – 500 mg per day

Ask in your health food shop if you need advice on dietary supplements

Dietary Recommendations

- Do not delay or miss meals
- Do not rely on snacks
- **Avoid:** alcohol, chocolate, cheese, citrus fruits, nuts meats, including sausages, dairy products, coffee and tea nitrate-containing foods MSG-containing foods, shellfish
- **Increase:** calcium- and magnesium-containing foods, oily fish

Guidelines for healthy eating

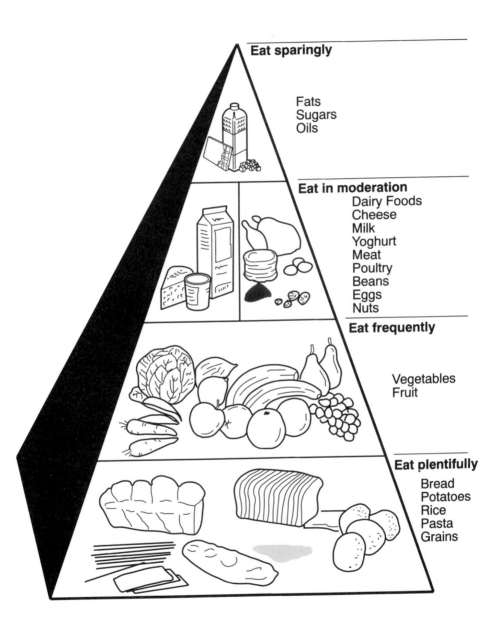

Eat sparingly

Fats
Sugars
Oils

Eat in moderation

Dairy Foods
Cheese
Milk
Yoghurt
Meat
Poultry
Beans
Eggs
Nuts

Eat frequently

Vegetables
Fruit

Eat plentifully

Bread
Potatoes
Rice
Pasta
Grains

The Healthy Eating Pyramid was evolved by nutritionists in the US. It has been adapted by the Dunn Nutritional Centre for application in Britain. It shows very clearly which foods we should be eating in large quantities and which we should be eating in only small amounts.

Elimination Diet

An allergy-free diet has two components: the identification of specific food allergens in the diet, and thereafter the allergen-free maintenance of the individual's diet on a day-to-day basis.

To identify the allergy-inducing foods, an elimination, or avoidance, diet is begun. Once the offending foods are identified, the maintenance diet can be designed.

What Is An Elimination Diet?

The elimination diet is an important diagnostic tool for food allergies. To begin the elimination diet, leave out the following common allergens from the diet for a period of 2 weeks: milk, eggs, wheat, sugar (both sugar cane and beet sugar), corn, citrus fruits, chocolate, coffee, additives, preservatives and food colourings.

If symptoms decrease or disappear with the omission of all these items, foods can be added back at the rate of a food item a day until the causes and symptoms of the food allergies are identified. If symptoms persist even after several weeks of eating only the foods that are allowed on the elimination diet, then each 'allowed' food needs to tested individually for its allergenicity.

Beginning The Elimination Diet

Here are some guidelines to help you begin the elimination diet:
- Before starting this diet, get a doctor's or a health-care professional's approval. It is also good to inquire about guidelines for taking medications, as *antihistamines* (drugs used in the treatment of allergies) may sometimes mask allergic reactions.
- Start a food diary. Use the diary for writing down everything you eat throughout the day. Also, use the diary for recording the appearance of symptoms and the time(s) when they occur. The food diary is a crucial part of the elimination diet.
- Look through cookery books for recipes using ingredients you know you can tolerate and use a few recipes to create menus that are appetising. Patient compliance can be improved if the entire family participates in the diet.
- After menus are developed, create a detailed grocery list. When first shopping for allergy-free foods, allow extra time for reading labels and finding substitute ingredients.

- A health-food store owner may know of acceptable food sources or might be able to order certain foods specially. In some cases, wheat-free foods may be available on prescription from your doctor.
- The diet should be followed for at least 2 to 3 weeks in order for you to become symptom-free. This is because allergens of previously eaten foods may remain in the body for one or more weeks.
- It is extremely important to remember that eating even a small amount of the allergenic food can produce symptoms, so do not deviate from the diet thinking that 'It won't hurt to have just a taste'. If the allergenic food is eaten accidentally, continue with the diet. However, stay on the diet for 2 to 3 weeks more from the date you ate the suspected allergen. Do not become discouraged since this happens to almost everyone!
- Do not forget that simply inhaling the odours of some foods can cause allergic symptoms in very sensitive people.

Testing Foods For Allergenicity

Once allergy symptoms disappear, add foods back to the diet one at a time to see which ones produce reactions.

To test a food, for instance sweet corn, eliminate it in all forms for 3 weeks. Then eat increasing amounts of pure sweet corn, such as corn on the cob, flaked corn or maize grits, for 3 consecutive days. On the first day, eat a small amount (such as 1 serving of corn flakes) and eat a larger portion on the following days. If allergic symptoms develop, stop eating the sweet corn immediately.

If allergic symptoms do not develop, you can probably assume that sweet corn is acceptable. Thus, continue to eat sweet corn while the next suspected allergen is tested in the same manner. Wait 3 days before introducing a new food since a delayed reaction to sweet corn may occur. Continue recording the foods eaten and any symptoms which may occur.

When an allergy-provoking food is identified, check the *biological classification* of that food. Sensitivity to one item in a food class indicates the possibility of a cross-reaction with another item listed under the same category. For example, if you are allergic to wheat, you may also be allergic to other members of the grain family, such as corn, rye, barley, etc. Test each related food separately. A proven food allergen may be reintroduced into the diet after several months. If symptoms reappear, avoid the food for several more months. If no

symptoms recur, add the food back into your diet, eating it only once every few days or weeks to avoid redevelopment of the allergy.

Finding A Nutrition Therapist

For a list of practitioners or further information write, enclosing a SAE to:

The British Naturopathic and Osteopathic Association, 6 Netherall Gardens, London NW3 5 RR;

The British Society for Nutritional Medicine, 4 Museum Street, York, YO1 2ES;

The Nutrition Association, 36 Wycombe Road, Marlow, Buckinghamshire SL7 3HX;

The Nutrition Consultants Association, c/o The Institute of Optimum Nutrition, 5 Jerdan Street, London SW6 1BE;

The Society for the Promotion of Nutritional Therapy, First Floor, The Enterprise Centre, Station Parade, Eastbourne BN1 1BE.

Further Reading

Migraine and Epilepsy by Jan De Vries (Mainstream Publishing)
Migraine – Special Diets Cook Books by Celia Norman (Thorsons)
Naturopathic Medicine by Roger Newman Turner (Thorsons)
The Migraine Revolution by Dr John Mansfield (Thorsons)
Vitamin Guide by Hasnain Walji (Element Books)
Vitamins, Minerals and Dietary Supplements: A Definitive Guide by Hasnain Walji (Headway)

HERBAL MEDICINE: BACK TO BASICS

According to the World Health Organisation (WHO), herbalism is three to four times more commonly practised than conventional medicine. This may seem rather a surprising statement since renewed interest in herbal medicine in the West is relatively recent. However, in the East herbalism is widely used and it is evident that the healing power of herbs has been a source of curing disease and illness from the earliest civilisations.

In ancient times, food and medicine were inextricably linked and food was eaten for its health-giving properties as well as its taste. The Romans and Egyptians were particularly adept at using herbs and it is known that the builders of the pyramids took a daily ration of garlic to preserve their health and to ward off infections. Chinese and Indian peoples also relied heavily on herbal medicine and it still plays an important part in medical practice to this day. Herbal preparations form part of Indian Ayurvedic medicine and in China there are numerous schools of herbalism and herbal dispensaries can be found in most hospitals.

In the West, herbs were used in everyday life and in medieval times all monasteries cultivated herb gardens. Monks were often considered to be knowledgeable in medical matters and their advice was sought for a whole variety of ailments. With the development of the printing press in the fifteenth century, there was a surge in the number of herbal compilations and publications and many herbalists set up their own apothecary shops. Later, herbal medicine took on a more global character as herbs from Europe, the Middle East, Asia and the Americas were used in conjunction and in combination with each other. Advances in navigation and international travel made this possible.

In 1864, a number of herbalists founded the National Association (later Institute) of Medical Herbalists which, in its early days and to this day, has had to resist attempts from orthodox medical pressure groups who wanted the practice of herbal medicine banned. Recently, the resurgence of interest in herbal medicine has

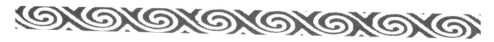

coincided with increased general concern for ecology and the environment. The perceived safer approach of using herbal remedies for common ailments especially, has also contributed to its new-found popularity and many herbal preparations can now be bought over the counter.

In fact, orthodox medicine developed from herbal medicine. Many synthesised drugs have their origins in plant material. Aspirin was first extracted from the medicinal herbs meadowsweet and black willow. Many steroids are now synthesised from a chemical first extracted from the Mexican wild yam. The medical profession regards plants and herbs as a source of active chemical ingredients which are then extracted and later synthesised to become potent drugs, some of which have produced notorious side-effects in their synthesised form.

A Holistic Approach

Herbalists believe that the drug companies' search for the 'active ingredients' in plants, which are then isolated and synthesised to make medicines, is a misguided approach. They maintain that the whole plant offers a safer and more effective treatment than artificially combined constituents which may be more powerful and, as a result, considerably more dangerous.

Another difference between herbal medicine and orthodox medicine is that in herbalism good health is regarded as being more than simply absence of disease. Rather, it is a state of positive well-being. So herbal medicine aims not just to relieve the symptoms of a disease but actively to seek out the true cause of a problem, often by creating the correct conditions that encourage the body to heal itself.

Herbalism recognises the mental or spiritual aspects of a health problem as well as the physical; the social and economic conditions that perpetuate ill-health are also acknowledged. Treatment, unlike that prescribed by conventional medicine, is tailored to meet the particular needs of the individual.

What Is A Herb?

To most people, herbs are plants used in cooking to add flavour, or they are ingredients in cosmetics, or home remedies for medicinal purposes. To a botanist, a herb is a nonwoody plant under the

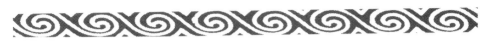

height of 30 cm, whereas, to a gardener, herbs are ornamental plants used in a herbaceous border. However, to a medical herbalist, a herb is any plant material – including seeds, bark, flowers, and even ferns, mosses, fungi and seaweed – that can be used in medicine and health care.

The term 'herbal medicine' covers a very wide range of uses of plants, for example, in naturopathy and aromatherapy, as well as simple herbal medicine. Even within herbalism there are many different types of prescription. Western medical herbalists usually use a combination of herbs for a specific condition, although some simple single herbs are also prescribed. In other systems, especially the Chinese, herbal preparations are made in carefully formulated combinations.

You can buy the herbal equivalent of fast food, the over-the-counter tablet. But herbal remedies can also be taken in the form of *tisanes* and teas prepared by infusing the plant material in hot water. Herbal baths are another alternative. Medication can even take the form of syrups or extraction drops to be held under the tongue, where they can be absorbed quickly through the mucous tissues. Steam inhalation is a further option. Externally, herbs may be applied in the form of compresses, creams and ointments. For further information, see *Headway Lifeguides: Herbalism,* by Frances Büning and Paul Hambly.

How Does Herbal Medicine Work?

Herbal medicines are thought to trigger off *neurochemical* (the body's nervous and chemical) responses which are a natural part of the healing process. By taking herbal medication in moderate doses over a period of time, these biochemical responses become automatic, even when the medication is discontinued.

The herbal formulas (as the compound medicines are known) fulfil three basic functions: to eliminate and cleanse as laxatives, diuretics and as blood purifiers; as relaxants or tonics, working on the nervous system; to nourish and restore weakened or exhausted tissues.

Herbal remedies are medicines and need to be treated with respect. Taking excessive doses can be harmful to your health. Nevertheless, herbal medicine, if used sensibly, is generally recognised as being far safer than conventional medicine; mainly because, in taking the whole plant, the dosage level of active ingredients is kept low.

Using Herbs

Herbs need not be taken as a medicine but can be included in the daily diet as a means of keeping healthy and clearing up minor ailments. For example, one of the most valuable herbs is garlic and it can be consumed fresh or included in food to add a distinctive flavour. It is also possible to make herbal drinks at home by putting a heaped teaspoon of a herb in a cup of boiling water and leaving it to steep for 4 to 5 minutes. Other ways of taking herbs in liquid form are:

- *Decoction:* for preparations made from roots and bark. Put a heaped tablespoon of powdered dried herb into a stainless steel (not aluminium) saucepan, with a pint of boiling water, bring to the boil and allow to simmer for 10 to 15 minutes. Strain and drink.
- *Infusion:* fresh or dried herbs may be used in loose or tea-bag form. The method is to warm a teapot and put in a dessertspoon of herb for each cup required. Pour in a cup of boiling water for each cup required and allow to steep for 10 to 15 minutes.
- *Tincture:* an alcohol-based concentrated preparation to be taken in small doses.
- *Tisane:* sold as tea-bags and made with boiling water, to be drunk straight away without lengthy steeping.

Herbs can be obtained from fresh food shops or may be found growing in the wild or in your garden. If you do decide to collect wild herbs you should take note of the following points:

- Ensure that the area you harvest has not been sprayed with chemical fertilisers or that it is close to a public highway where it may have been contaminated by car exhaust fumes.
- You need to be sure of the particular plant you are picking. Some varieties of plant are similar in appearance, so a good book on flora should accompany you on your expedition.
- Do not pick a plant that is uncommon; ensure that the plant is not a protected species – it is fine to pick nettles, but not to pick cowslip flower. Alternatively, a herb garden can be cultivated, as most herbs are relatively easy to grow and cuttings are available at most garden centres.

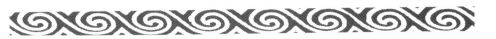

Western Herbal Remedies

Headaches

Stress is considered to be the most common catalyst for transforming painless muscle tension into a headache, so herbs are often prescribed for the easing of the muscle tension itself.

Useful herbs include melissa, cayenne, chamomile, elderflower, Jamaican dogwood, marjoram, peppermint, rosemary, rose, skullcap, thyme, valerian, wood betony and wormwood.

Herbal Remedies for Headaches

A suggested combination of herbs for headaches and nervous problems follows:

> Catnip – herb – 1 part
> Valerian – root – 1 part
> Lemon verbena – herb – 1 part
> Skullcap – herb – 1 part
> Take as a tea, made by infusing the herbs for 10 to 15 minutes, up to 3 times a day.
>
> **For a stomach-related headache try the following tea:**
> Cold balm – 1 part
> Lavender – 1 part
> Meadowsweet – 1 part
> To be taken as an infusion, steeped for 10 to 15 minutes.
>
> **For a headache related to menstrual problems:**
> Skullcap – 1 part
> Valerian – 1 part
> Take as an infusion, steeped for 10 to 15 minutes

Migraine

Common triggers are stress and diet, although for an effective cure specific causes need to be identified. Lavender and feverfew are generally considered to be the most beneficial herbs for migraine.

Herbalists consider it important to distinguish between 'hot' and 'cold' types of migraine:

- **Cold migraines** involve excess *vasodilation* (widening of blood vessels, causing increased blood flow) where the application of cold packs is relieving. These kind of migraines are helped by circulatory stimulants.
- **Hot migraines** involve excessive *vasoconstriction* (narrowing of blood vessels, causing reduced blood flow) and are helped by a prescription that emphasises bitter, relaxant or sedative remedies.

In addition, eliminative remedies, such as laxatives, should be considered if there is a digestive disorder.

To ease the pain of attack in the initial stages of migraine, the following herbs are beneficial: black willow, Jamaican dogwood, passion flower, valerian and wood betony.

For digestive symptoms, such as nausea and vomiting, black horehound, chamomile, golden seal and meadowsweet are useful.

Chinese Herbal Remedies

Chinese herbalists, like Western herbalists, treat headaches with specific herb remedies which are non habit-forming. Before prescribing any herbs, a practitioner will take the patient's pulse. Over the centuries, the method of taking a pulse has been developed into a sophisticated form of diagnosis. With the right hand the herbalist feels the patient's left pulse, and with the left hand he/she feels the right pulse. Placing the index, middle and ring finger over the pulse, he/she applies varying degrees of pressure. The position of the finger and the amount of pressure applied reveal the condition of the various organs, such as the stomach, liver, intestine and gall-bladder. The Chinese consider that the action of the *yin* and *yang* – the two opposing and dual forces that that regulate the universe – also manifest themselves in the body and that all diseases are a result of a disturbed harmony between *yin* and *yang* in the body. Chinese herbalists contend that herbs are substances which have life, and help the body in harmonising the *yin* and *yang*.

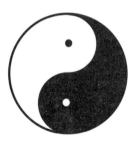

The yin-yang symbol

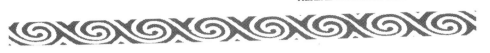

For nervous headaches *Chi-hsueh-ts'ao* (catnip), which belongs the the mint family, is useful. Usually this is combined with other herbs, such as valerian, celery seeds and oats, and prepared as a tea. Another remedy for headaches is *Lu-Ts'ao* (hops).

Ma-pien-ta'ao (vervain) is a particularly effective remedy for tension or congestive headaches as well as migraine. Usually, simple vervain tea will bring relief from migraines. But a more effective treatment is a decoction of vervain, dandelion root, ginger root, marshmallow root, motherwort, wild carrot and centuary. This, taken for several weeks, will reduce the number and severity of what the Chinese term 'liverish migraine'. Liver trouble is considered the commonest cause of migraine. The theory is that normally the bile that forms in the liver is thin and clear and flows freely through the gall-bladder ducts to empty the bladder periodically. However, if the bile thickens, due to the ingestion of foods that cause congestion of the bile ducts, and the flow is impaired, the gall-bladder does not empty completely. This build-up of bile is believed to be a cause of migraine. So long as the bile is not eliminated, headache and nausea will persist. A Chinese herbalist will advise the patient to drink a glass or two of plain hot water to get the bile flowing and to continue drinking glasses of water every couple of hours until excess bile is eliminated. This water treatment may relieve the condition but will not prevent future attacks. The answer is to reduce fatty and indigestible foods and to take the vervain decoction 3 times a day before meals.

Mi-Tieh-Hsiang (rosemary) prepared as tea is also reputed to be particularly useful for simple headaches. Another method for using rosemary for prompt relief of congestive headaches is to hold a small bottle of spirits of rosemary close to the the nose and inhale the fumes. A few drops rubbed gently on the forehead and the temples may also help.

Consulting A Medical Herbalist

A medical herbalist can give more specialist advice on the use of herbal medicine for serious or long-term problems. Medical herbalists undergo a four-year course at the School of Herbal Medicine and are trained to carry out full medical examinations. At an initial consultation a practitioner will ask the patient for details of his/her medical history, eating and exercise habits and whether stress is a factor in daily life. As a result of the overall diagnosis, the

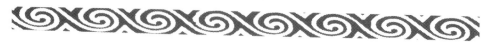

herbalist will prescribe a single herb or combination of herbs and specify in which form the medicine is to be taken, such as a tincture, as pills or as infusions.

Practitioners are usually members of the National Institute of Medical Herbalists and apply Western herbal medicine in a consulting room. The diagnostic techniques of many qualified medical herbalists resemble those of GPs, using the same methods and equipment for blood pressure, pulse taking, physical examination and assessment of urine and blood samples.

Write to the National Institute of Medical Herbalists, 9 Palace Gate, Exeter EX1 1JA for a list of medical herbalists.

Chinese Herbalists

Traditional Chinese herbalists tend to be confined to Chinese centres, practising mainly within the Chinese community. 'Modern' practitioners of Chinese herbalism often use herbs in conjunction with acupuncture.

Write to the Register of Chinese Herbal Medicine, 138 Prestbury Road, Cheltenham GLS2 2DP for information.

Ayurvedic And Unani Practitioners

Commonly known as *Vaids* and *Hakims*, these practitioners are mainly found within the Indian and Pakistani communities and offer treatment based on traditional principles.

Further Reading

A–Z of Modern Herbalism by Simon Mills (Diamond Books)
Herbal First Aid by Andrew Chevallier (Amberwood)
Herbal Medicine by Dian Dincin Buchman (Rider Books)
Herbalism: Headway Lifeguides by Francis Büning and Paul
    Hambly (Headway)
Natural Healing with Herbal Combination by B Wright
Potter's New Cyclopaedia of Botanical Drugs by R C Wren (C W Daniel)
Thorsons' Guide to Medical Herbalism by David Hoffman (Thorsons)
Traditional Home Herbal Remedies by Jan de Vries (Mainstream
    Publishing)

5

HOMOEOPATHY: A DIFFERENT PERSPECTIVE ON SYMPTOMS

Homoeopathy is based on the natural law *Similia similibus curentur*, which means 'Like cures like'. In other words, a disease can be cured by giving a substance which, if given to a healthy person, produces effects similar to the symptoms of that disease.

Homoeopathy is a holistic therapy which aims to go beyond the mere alleviation of symptoms to address the actual causes of ill-health. The ultimate aim of homoeopathic medicine is for the patient to reach such a level of health that there is no longer a need for, or dependence on, any medicine or therapy.

The therapy has its roots in ancient times. Homoeopathic principles are present in the writings of the fifth-century Greek physician Hippocrates, while the sixteenth-century Swiss alchemist Paracelsus commented that, 'Those who merely study and treat the effects of disease are like those who imagine that they can drive away winter by brushing snow from the door. It is not the snow that causes the winter but the winter that causes the snow.' Symptoms are not actually manifestations of a disease but rather the attempts of the body to heal itself.

Modern homoeopathy owes its establishment to the German physician Samuel Hahnemann. As a doctor in the late eighteenth and early nineteenth centuries, he was appalled at the way conventional medicine was practised. He considered the customs of bleeding patients, administering strong enemas and using powerful, and often dangerous, drugs to be both brutal and dangerous, evidenced by the high patient death-rate.

Hahnemann searched for a method of curing that was effective, safe and gentle. While translating Cullen's *Materia Medica*, Hahnemann was puzzled by the explanation for the efficacy of cinchona bark in treating malaria. He proceeded to dose himself liberally with cinchona bark for several days and developed malarial symptoms. In this way he established that, not only did cinchona

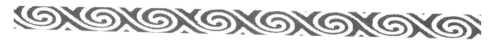

bark alleviate the intermittent fever of malaria, but large doses of cinchona bark actually caused malarial symptoms in a normally healthy person.

Hahnemann went on to experiment with many other substances, testing them on himself, his family and friends. These experiments, called 'provings', involved the taking of very small doses of substances and carefully noting all the symptoms that were produced. Subsequently, patients suffering from similar symptoms were treated with the 'proven' substances; the results were encouraging and often remarkable.

Hahnemann's research led him to criticise conventional medicine, especially *allopathic treatment* (orthodox treatment of an illness with its opposite). Instead, he argued, the remedy for the healing of the disease should be one that artificially produces symptoms as similar as possible to those produced by the disease itself; 'Like cures like.'

The theory of homoeopathy developed, although not without opposition from the orthodox medical profession. Its value was particularly highlighted in the European cholera epidemics when many lives were saved by a homoeopathic prescription of camphor suggested by Hahnemann. By the time of Hahnemann's death in 1843, homoeopathy had spread over most of continental Europe and had penetrated Russia, South America, Great Britain and parts of the USA.

How Homoeopathy Works

The fundamental difference between homoeopathic and allopathic medicine lies in the way in which symptoms are viewed. While allopathic medicine views symptoms as being part of the disease, a homoeopath regards them as an adaptive response by the body in defending itself. Simply put, the symptoms are evidence of the body's fight against the disease. The homoeopath's task is to prescribe a remedy that will stimulate the body to heal itself more quickly. The correct remedy is one that will create symptoms similar to those of the disease process as presented by the patient.

Homoeopathy is based on the following three principles:

The Law Of Similars

The human organism is believed to have a great capacity to heal itself and is in a constant state of self-repair. The homoeopath

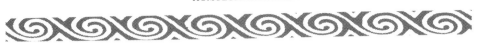

prescribes a remedy which, through previous 'provings' on healthy people and from clinical observations, is known to produce a similar symptom picture to that of the patient. The prescribed remedy then stimulates and assists the body's own natural healing efforts.

The Single Remedy

Homoeopaths believe that the body should only be stimulated by a single remedy at any one time. It is the patient's whole system which is out of balance even though there may be a multiplicity of symptoms which may not appear to be connected. The single remedy allows the homoeopath clearly to observe and evaluate its effect before further prescription is considered.

The Minimal Dose

Only a minute dose, in the form of a specially prepared potency, is needed, since the patient is highly sensitive to its stimulus. This is because of the similarity between the remedy's known symptom picture and that of the patient. The specific potency and number of doses are determined by the homoeopath according to the needs of the individual.

Much debate and controversy surrounds the concept of dilution. As homoeopathic remedies are diluted to such an extent, sceptics say that it is inconceivable that any of the original substance is left at all, so how can such a remedy work? Homoeopaths would argue that, although they do not yet understand the mechanism, there is ample evidence that it does work.

Theories And Clinical Trials

Among the wide range of theories put forward to explain how homoeopathy works, one is the suggestion that looking for a physical explanation ignores the holistic nature of the therapy. It may well be the case that the high potencies are acting at a very subtle level of energy, as with *chi* in Chinese medicine or *prana* in Ayurvedic medicine, and that these remedies vibrate or resonate with a person's 'vital force'. The right homoeopathic remedy is like a boost of subtle energy which returns the body to its optimum frequency and so aids recovery. Once the body is in tune, resonating at its appropriate rate, it is able to use its immune system to throw off the negative stimuli that cause illness.

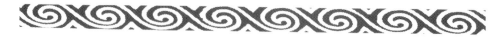

There were many clinical trials in the late 1970s. One in particular, conducted in Glasgow in 1978, compared three groups of patients with rheumatoid arthritis. One group was told to take aspirin, another group a *placebo* (a non-medicated substance) and the last group homoeopathic medicines. A year after the commencement of the trial, the condition in the homoeopathic group was more significantly improved than in the two other groups.

Other trials conducted since then include David Reilly and Morag Taylor's hay fever trial in 1985, and Peter Fisher's fibrositis trial in 1986. In both of these, homoeopathic medicines were found to have a demonstrable effect in relieving symptoms. A recent study of over 100 clinical trials showed about 80 positive in favour of homoeopathic medicines.

The Homoeopathic Medicines

The range of sources for homoeopathic medicines is immense, since they can be prepared from anything that causes symptoms. Most come from plants but some come from metals and minerals. Today there are over 2,500 substances that have been prepared for homoeopathic medicines, from belladonna (deadly nightshade) and aconite (monkshood) to lachesis (an extract of snake venom) and cantharis (derived from the insect known as Spanish fly).

The medicines are made up by taking the raw material through a process of serial dilution and *succussion* (vigorous shaking). Each stage of succussion increases the potency, or strength, which is given a number and a letter. Potencies with an 'X' affix are diluted 1:9 and those with a 'C' affix are diluted 1:99 at each successive stage. Plant materials are instantly soluble, but minerals and metals need to undergo a process called *trituration* (grinding) with a milk/sugar powder up to the 3X potency before they become soluble; at that point the dilution and succession process continues in the same manner as plants.

Taking The Medicines

The remedy and potency prescribed are matched to the needs and vitality of the patient and also to the vitality of the disease process of the patient. The potency has to be similar in resonance to that of the disease, as well as similar to the symptom picture. Today there are many outlets which sell homoeopathic medicines over the counter,

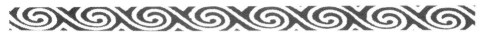

such as health food stores and pharmacies. They are available in tablet form, granules, pilules, powders or as a liquid, while there are creams, ointments and lotions for external use. It is usual for over-the-counter medicines to be of a lower potency, either 6C or 30C – caution is advised in the repetition of the 30C, as this is a relatively high potency. Higher potency medicines are generally recommended for use only by experienced and qualified homoeopaths.

The same medicine may be administered in different ways, perhaps a single dose in a high-potency form or a low dose repeated frequently. The choice of method depends on the nature of the illness and the individual needs of the patient. For example, if a person has been ill for a long time and the body is in physical disrepair, one way to take the homoeopathic medicine would be in repeated doses in a lower potency to stimulate the immune system. However, a healthier person may just need a single high-potency remedy for a response.

Dilution lessens the toxic effects of the substance used; this contrasts markedly with the powerful drugs often used in allopathic medicine, a number of which have been known to produce alarming side-effects. Further, since conventional drugs are prescribed for their individual capacities to work upon specific parts of the body, it follows that several different drugs might be prescribed to treat various symptoms in one individual. The effects of such combinations are often unknown or not recognised. A homoeopath, however, prescribes a single medicine in an appropriate potency which will stimulate a person's immune or defence mechanism and bring about an improvement in general health.

Headaches And Migraine

The most appropriate medicine for your problem will be chosen on an individual basis; in other words, your homoeopath will be looking for the symptoms that are specific to you. So he/she will be asking questions that make it clear, through a process of elimination, that one kind of remedy is more appropriate for you at this particular time than another kind. Thus, for example, you may be asked whether your headache is worse when you are lying down or whether it is affected by hot or cold weather, and if you are an irritable or weepy person. Descriptions for some of the remedies follow:

Headaches

- *Arsenicum album:* for a burning, throbbing headache where the discomfort is briefly eased by placing a cold, damp flannel on the head (although Arsenicum is usually associated with being better for hot applications, in the case of headaches it could be alleviated by cold applications or cool, fresh air); when pains cause anxiety and restlessness; when vomiting and nausea are present; when it is made worse from noise, movement and light, and eased by lying propped up on pillows in a dark room.
- *Belladonna:* for use when the headache is violent or throbbing and the pain is momentarily eased by pressing on the head and sitting up; when the pain worsens in the event of any sudden movement, jarring, stooping, sudden noise or strong light; better from cold applications and in some cases, fresh air; when there is a sensitive scalp with headache, worse from getting hair wet, cold on head and even from cutting hair – often sudden onset of symptoms.
- *Chamomilla:* use for a bursting, one-sided headache which is worsened by cold and may be eased by warmth which causes the sufferer to be irritable. The headache may be brought on by anger or drinking too much coffee and gets worse in the evening.
- *Bryonia:* for use when a bursting, splitting headache is worse for least movement and better for cool air, and is eased by steady pressure and lying motionless; when worse for warmth in any form, and after meals; when it may be accompanied by constipation.
- *Kali bich:* for a dull, heavy headache with the pain in small areas or over one eye and accompanied by catarrh; for sinus headaches; when pains are worse between 2 – 3 a.m. and from motion, and better for warmth.
- *Gelsemium:* use when the headache is heavy and dull and there is pain in the neck, blurred vision and giddiness; when the pain spreads from the neck to the forehead above the eyes; when there is a feeling of a tight band around the head; when it is better for profuse urination and worse from hot rooms, tiredness and anticipatory anxiety.
- *Nux vomica:* for a heavy headache which is worse for excitement and in cold or noise; for hangover headaches – often with constipation; when it is better for a short sleep or being left undisturbed; very irritable, becoming angry and impatient with pain. Worse from unwanted attention.
- *Euphrasia:* for a bursting headache with painful, watery eyes where the sufferer is unable to bear bright light. Catarrhal headache often accompanied with discharge from eyes and nose.

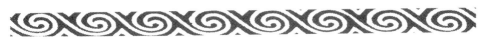

- *Kali phos:* use where the headache is accompanied by a humming in the ears; when pain present on waking; sensation of a band around the forehead. Better for gentle motion. Always hungry with headache.
- *Pulsatilla:* for a pulsating or bursting headache associated with digestive upsets from rich food; worse for warm, stuffy rooms and keeping still; better for cool applications and walking in fresh air; also from gentle movement; when you are weepy and in need of sympathy when in pain.
- *Sepia:* for a severe one-sided headache with shooting pain which is relieved by a long sleep or vigorous movement in the fresh air; when there is terrible nausea with sensitivity to cooking smells, light and noise.

Migraine

Migraine is a chronic condition and patients should seek professional advice if the self-help treatment does not produce a positive effect.

- *Iris versicolor:* use for dull throbbing or shooting pain on the right side of the forehead; when there is blurring of vision before the onset of the headache, nausea and/or the scalp feels tight; when there is sick pain often brought on by eating too many sweet things; when there is salivation with pain; when you are constipated before, or during migraine.
- *Natrum Muriaticum:* for a throbbing and burning head and tingling, or when numbness in the face signals an attack, which is preceded by misty vision or zig-zag lines; for headaches with travel sickness and pallor; when better for lying down and after sleep and worse when moving eyes.
- *Sanguinaria:* for a right-sided headache which starts at the back of the head and extends upwards and settles over the eyes, especially the right eye – accompanied by shivering and nausea and is better for vomiting; when it is much worse from jolting or jarring or any noise; when pains are relieved by sleep; when attacks often start in the morning and improve by the evening.
- *Spigelia:* for a left-sided headache burning like hot needles made worse by bending or movement, with palpitations and pounding in the head; the eye waters on the affected side; the neck may feel numb and the back of the head may be tender; hypersensitive to pain and touch.
- *Kali bich:* use where there is blurring of vision with nausea before the migraine. These symptoms may improve as the headache increases; when pain is worse at night and for cold, stooping or walking; localised pain from suppressed catarrh; when you must lie down with pain; where

there are sharp, shooting, shifting pains that are worse waking from sleep and better for warmth and firm pressure.

- *Lachesis:* for left-sided bursting pain which carries on after sleep and is made worse from sunlight; pains are throbbing and may extend from the left eye to the root of the nose; pains are relieved by lying down, open air or warmth; better for onset of discharges – catarrh or menstruation; pains extending to neck and shoulders.

A Conversation With A Practitioner

Q. What are the goals of homoeopathic treatment?

A. The goal is to get you to a level of health, balance and freedom from limitations so that you eventually need only very infrequent medication.

Q. Why do homoeopaths ask so many questions?

A. Constitutional homoeopathy does not treat specific diseases as such, but treats individuals. Hence a detailed understanding of the patient is fundamental to making a correct prescription.

The homoeopath must attempt an almost impossible task – that of coming quickly to a complete understanding of an individual. The questioning process is essential for forming and developing this understanding.

The homoeopath needs to be an acute listener and observer – our job is primarily to get your symptom picture and to match this to a remedy. So we want to hear your story and listen sympathetically, without making any value judgements, and match this information to the right remedy.

To match a remedy to an individual we must know all the person's limitations clearly: this includes mental, emotional and physical levels, and such aspects as general energy, effects of environment and causative factors.

Q. How many appointments are necessary?

A. In the beginning, that is, in the first six months, visits may be more frequent and will taper off as you become healthier. We feel we need to see you initially more frequently (follow-ups are usually every four-to-six weeks in the beginning) to work with you and evaluate your progress. Yet we are not insensitive to the cost of treatment and do not wish to make this a burden.

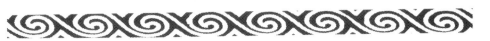

If a remedy has acted curatively, even in deep and complex cases, after the initial follow-up we may not need to see you for some time. This is because the remedy has brought your system into balance and, in our experience, this state can last for a long time. We also need to wait until the next 'remedy picture' comes up clearly. This is the time to have a renewed faith in your body's healing abilities.

Q. How can I be involved?

A. You don't have to believe in homoeopathic remedies in order for them to work (we treat babies and there are homoeopathic vets). But to select the correct remedy and for the treatment to continue to act, your co-operation and commitment is necessary.
You can help by:

- Noting any changes after you take the remedy – keeping a weekly journal can be helpful for bringing to your follow-up consultations. Please note general changes as well as specific ones.
- Giving a clear and complete account of your symptoms on all levels.
- Above all, communicating any concerns or questions you may have. We are always trying to find better ways of helping you and welcome your comments.

Q. How do homoeopaths evaluate a curative response?

A. Homoeopaths have, through over 170 years of experience, developed sophisticated means of evaluating curative responses and have established laws and principles of cure.
On a simpler level, you want to see the problems you have come with clear up, and they should. Always keep in mind that ours is a total perspective on you and we want to see overall improvements as well as specific ones. You also have to see improvement in the context of the amount of stress in your life. So improvements will occur on physical, emotional and mental levels, and in general energy. Observe and report these general changes as well as specific ones.

Q. How long does treatment take?

A. This is a difficult question to answer but after several interviews the homoeopath is better able to give you an idea of this. In simpler problems and in acute situations, results can begin quickly and dramatically.
For a small percentage of very healthy individuals, one or two treatments may be all that is needed to stabilise the system for years at a stretch but such an ideal would, for most people, be an unrealistic expectation.

Q. Should I come back after I am feeling better?

A. The four-to-six week follow-up is important to return for. After you are feeling consistently better we would like to see you for regular check-ups to prevent future problems. Usually this is at four-to-six month intervals.

Q. How can a few doses do anything or last a long time?

A. The remedies are highly potent – they are prepared in what is called a 'potentised' dilution and dropped on to tiny lactose granules, pilules, tablets or powders, or can be taken in liquid form. They simply catalyse or trigger a response by the body on an energetic level, rather than effect chemical change. So, ultimately, what works better after the remedy is taken is your own regulating system. The remedy helps the body develop a natural, positive momentum which continues to gain strength and eliminate disease.

Should you want to gain a more in-depth understanding of this fascinating and profound process, refer to any of the introductory books on homoeopathy.

Q. Is there any advice about diet and lifestyle?

A. The homoeopath doesn't always give advice about lifestyle and diet. A good diet is, of course, essential for a healthy body. Any advice about diet and exercise is tailored to the individual's own needs in terms of their illness, age, and various environmental factors. This is because we always want to see clearly whether the homoeopathic remedy alone is working. Also we believe that when the organism is healthy an imbalanced lifestyle will diminish and positive changes will permeate all aspects of your life. There may be obvious 'obstacles to cure' in your life or environment which the homoeopath will discuss with you.

Q. Can homoeopathy work in more complex or chronic cases, and how long does it take?

A. In more complex cases, homoeopathic treatment is like peeling away the layers of an onion. Briefly, this means that we build up layers of symptoms, or 'pathology' as a response to certain stresses as we go through life. These layers are laid down and can be peeled away effectively with homoeopathic remedies. During treatment, old sets of symptoms may come up (but because with each successive remedy you are healthier they will not be as severe as in the past). A recurrence of an old set of symptoms may be the indication for a new remedy to be given. Even some hereditary tendencies can be eliminated with homoeopathy. So in deep or chronic problems the curative process may be gradual and consultations more frequent.

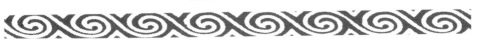

Q. What happens if the symptoms seem to return?

A. If you had a good curative response to a remedy and then after, say, two to six months (or at any time) a relapse seems to occur, we usually recommend waiting a few days to see if your system re-balances itself. If any severe symptoms develop, do not wait. If the symptoms persist after a week, then a repeat of the remedy or a follow-up remedy may be necessary. If so, another appointment would be needed.

Do not get disappointed or discouraged at this point and feel that homoeopathy is not working for you – this is just a phase of getting you to a consistently good state of health. This situation may mean a new remedy is indicated as a 'layer' of symptoms from the past comes up and needs to be treated.

Q. What will interfere with the remedy working?

A. Camphor products and highly aromatic essential oils, such as peppermint and menthol, can all interfere. There are certain therapies that can interfere, such as chemical therapies (natural or otherwise), high-potency vitamins, very intensive exercise programmes and certain dental procedures. It is not usually a good idea to have acupuncture during a course of homoeopathic treatment as it interferes with the 'vital force' and both treatments are based on the premise that they work by stimulating the body's healing powers.

We have found that massage, mild chiropractic and osteopathic treatments and certain gentle therapies or medications do not interfere with homoeopathy. If you are considering any other therapy, consult your homoeopath first. It is also best to avoid, or at least greatly reduce, the intake of stimulants such as coffee and other caffeine drinks.

Q. Can a wrong remedy be given and what are the effects?

A. As carefully as we try to match the correct remedy, we do not always achieve 100 per cent accuracy. If appropriately used, homoeopathic treatment should produce no side-effects from the remedies. Either nothing changes or the true symptom picture will become even clearer and the right remedy is more obvious.

It can take several interviews for a homoeopath to get an accurate picture of the totality of your symptoms and an 'essential' understanding of this in order to select the right remedy. Of course, the clearer and more in touch you are with yourself, the easier this task becomes.

Q. What about seeing a GP?

A. Homoeopathy is complementary to the health care that is available. We recommend that you should maintain your relationship with your

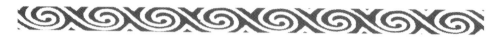

doctor, especially for routine needs and emergencies. Your GP will also arrange for you to have any blood tests or X-rays, etc. or refer you to a consultant.

Q. What about acute problems?
A. Homoeopathic remedies can treat acute problems such as flu and stomach upsets, and even help the body heal after injuries and falls. If you are already having homoeopathic treatment, mild illnesses will often clear up on their own, but if you are unsure or the symptoms are getting stronger, please phone for advice. If your symptoms are severe, phone immediately. If necessary contact your GP.

If you are involved in an accident or emergency you should go to your nearest casualty department for treatment and then phone to see if a homoeopathic remedy is also indicated.

Finding A Practitioner

An increasing number of qualified medical doctors now offer homoeopathic treatment. Most of them have taken a postgraduate training course to become a Member or a Fellow of the Faculty of Homoeopathy (MSHom or FFHom). A register of these is maintained by the Faculty of Homoeopathy, c/o Royal London Homoeopathic Hospital, Great Ormond Street, London WC1N 3HR. Many professional homoeopaths have trained for four years at accredited colleges and have become graduate or registered members of the Society of Homoeopaths (RSHom). For a list of registered homoeopaths, write to The Society of Homoeopaths, 2 Artizan Road, Northampton NN1 4HU.

In addition to the private and NHS practitioners, there are five NHS homoeopathic hospitals – London, Bristol, Tunbridge Wells, Liverpool and Glasgow. There are also a number of private clinics nationally. Further information about these may be obtained from The British Homoeopathic Association, 27A Devonshire Street, London W1N 1RJ.

Further Reading

Everybody's Guide to Homoeopathic Medicines by Stephen Cummings and Dana Ullman (Gollancz)
Homoeopathy for Babies And Children: A Parents' Guide by Beth MacEoin (Headway) publishing August, 1994

Homoeopathy for Emergencies by Phyllis Speight (C W Daniels)
Homoeopathy: Headway Lifeguides by Beth MacEoin
   (Headway)
Homoeopathy, Medicine for the New Man by George Vithoulkas
   (Thorsons)
Homoeopathy: Medicine for the 21st Century by Dana Ullman
   (Thorsons)
The Complete Homoeopathy Handbook: A Guide to Everyday Health Care
   by Miranda Castro (Macmillan)
*The Family Guide to Homoeopathy: The Safe Form of Medicine for the
   Future* by Andrew Lockie (Elm Tree Books)

6

ANTHROPOSOPHICAL MEDICINE: A BALANCED SYSTEM OF MEDICINE

The allopathic medical approach is based on a mechanistic view of the human being. In other words, it looks at the body rather than at the person. The growth of interest in other systems of medicine bears testimony to the fact that something is lacking.

Most of the alternative and complementary approaches to healing discussed in this book are based on ancient philosophies and the value systems of the civilisations that they represent. Anthroposophical practitioners, however, believe that turning to these in search of what is lacking in conventional medicine is like trying to turn the clock back. What is needed is not a return to the past, but an extension of conventional medicine to take account of both the spiritual and the physical sides of the person.

Anthroposophical medicine offers a spiritual dimension to allopathy. Its founder, the Austrian philosopher and scientist, Rudolf Steiner (1861–1925), sought to go beyond the limits of materialism in search of the spiritual side of human existence. He believed that we are made up of body, soul and spirit and anthroposophical medicine recognises that healing must take place on all levels. The foundations of anthroposophical medicine were laid when a Dutch doctor, Ita Wegman, in collaboration with Steiner, who was not a medical doctor himself, wrote a book called *The Fundamentals of Therapy* aimed at the medical profession. Anthroposophical medicine was to be regarded as an extension to conventional practice rather than as an alternative.

The Four Aspects Of A Complete Person

To the physical body must be added three other elements in order to complete the picture of a human being. In anthroposophical parlance, they are called the *etheric body, astral body* and *ego*. These nonmaterial elements are common to us all, but they cannot be

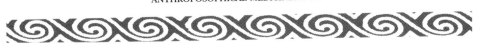

perceived with the physical senses. Sometimes the terms *life element,* *soul element* and *spirit*, respectively, are used. All these three nonphysical aspects maybe described as 'spiritual', but the spirit itself is the unique inner identity.

The Anthroposophical Elements Of A Complete Person			
Spirit	Self-consciousness	Human	Ego
Soul	Consciousness	Animal	Astral body
Life	Life	Plant	Etheric body
Material	Weighable and measurable	Mineral	Physical body

The Etheric Body

The etheric body, or the life element, can best be described as that force which governs the existence of the physical body. The best illustration of how the life element works is that after death the physical body, left under the influence of physical laws, begins to deteriorate from being a highly-organised structure into dust.

Not only is the etheric body responsible for building and organising growth, it is also responsible for maintaining and repairing parts of the physical body. It is this force that strives to keep us in good health and helps the physical body to recover from less serious ailments. The etheric body's continuous fight against death and decay in the physical body must be understood in order to comprehend fully any organism and its diseases.

The Astral Body

This soul element is what differentiates humans and animals from the plant kingdom. Both humans and animals are conscious of the physical world and have instinct. We all experience pain when the physical body is hurt, but we are also aware of inner pain when someone hurts our feelings. The main difference between anthroposophical doctors and conventional doctors is that the former consider the soul element as much as the physical element, while the latter rely principally on the physical.

The astral body has a *catabolic* (breaking down) effect on the physical body and, as such, has an opposite effect to the etheric body, which constantly strives to build and repair (*anabolic* effect). Anthroposophical practitioners believe that health prevails as long

as the destructive process, brought about by the astral body, is held in check by the building force of the etheric body. Any imbalance between these two forces will result in disease.

Ego

Awareness of the physical world and the experience of pleasure and pain are common characteristics of animals and human beings, because they both have astral bodies. Human beings have one additional level of consciousness that animals lack. It is the ability to think, together with an awareness that they are independent, conscious beings. Anthroposophical medicine describes this as the spirit, or the ego. This dimension has a dual effect on the physical body. It works with the etheric body in its anabolic activity, and with the astral body in its catabolic activity.

The Anthroposophical View Of Illness

Anthroposophical medicine looks at illness in terms of the interrelationships between the ego, the astral body, the etheric body and the physical body. It seeks to influence the activity of one or more of these elements so as to restore balance and, therefore, health.

The three main functional organ systems within anthroposophical medicine are described as the nerve–sense system, the metabolic limb system and the rhythmic system.

Associated with consciousness, the *nerve–sense system* incorporates the nerves, the brain, the spinal cord and the sense organs.

The *metabolic limb system* includes the stomach, intestines and the lymphatic system. This system is characterised by unconsciousness; we are not aware of its anabolic processes unless there is something wrong and we feel pain.

In the middle of these two is the *rhythmic system,* which is centred on the heart and the lungs. The rhythmic system plays a major role in the maintenance of health as it is involved in keeping the nerve–sense and the metabolic limb systems in a state of balance.

An excess in the activity of the metabolic limb system means an increase in warmth and an excess of fluid. Too much nerve–sense activity is characterised by a loss of fluid, excessive hardening, etc, which are all features of degenerative diseases. In fact, the anthroposophical system of medicine describes two main types of

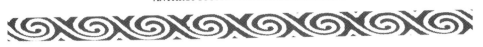

illness: inflammatory or feverish on the one hand, and degenerative and hardening on the other. It follows that when illness comes about as a result of an imbalance between the nerve–sense system and the metabolic limb system, healing can only be effected when the balance is restored. The practitioner uses different methods to achieve this.

The Three Systems In Anthroposophical Medicine

Nerve–Sense:	Thinking	Conscious	Cooling Catabolic Hardening
Rhythmic:	Feeling	Dream-like	Balancing Mediating
Metabolic Limb:	Volition	Unconscious	Warming Anabolic Softening

Use Of Medicines

The anthroposophical doctor looks for examples in nature and bases his/her remedies on natural life processes which are similar to those in the human organism. In contrast with conventional medicine, which analyses disease in terms of molecular change and develops medicine to counteract those changes so as to alleviate the symptoms, anthroposophical medicine looks at the interplay of the processes that cause the molecular changes associated with the symptoms.

Artistic Therapies

Based on the premise that artistic activities have an impact on the consciousness of an individual, as well as society as a whole, anthroposophical practitioners have devised a number of techniques that help in healing, such as music, painting, sculpture and architecture. Music, for example, which has a powerful impact on feelings, is an expression of the laws of the spirit within the realm of the soul. In other words, the ego is expressed at the astral level. Similarly, painting is an expression of the astral in the etheric realm, and sculpture a manifestation of the etheric level in the physical body. Rudolf Steiner devised an art of movement called *eurhythmy* to

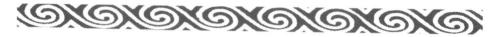

express the forms of movement of the etheric body in the physical realm.

Painting therapy has a wide range of indications, including the treatment of a number of disorders of the rhythmic system, such as asthma, in which the rhythm of breathing is impaired because the airways have been partially blocked. An anthroposophical practitioner would view this as the result of an imbalance between the airy and the watery elements, which correspond to the astral and etheric bodies respectively, and would seek to redress the balance.

Hydrotherapy And Massage

Water is the one medium that we have all experienced before birth in the womb and is therefore considered by practitioners to play a special role in the healing process. History illustrates the value placed on therapeutic baths by ancient civilisations and in the development of spa towns, many of which are still in existence today.

Baths with certain essential oils are helpful for the alleviation of circulatory and muscular problems and can distribute warmth where it may be lacking as a result of illness.

The therapeutic value of massage is well known. Anthroposophical medicine has developed a particular kind of massage known as *Rhythmic Massage* which aims to balance the etheric force with the tension created by the astral influence. This is done by encouraging regularity in breathing and heart action and the other cycles in order to harmonise the workings of bodily functions.

Headaches And Migraines

Tension headaches may be relieved by rhythmical massage where the masseur will vigorously knead the calves and feet. The theory is that, by causing spasm in the lower part of the body, excess astral activity will be diverted, thus bringing immediate relief. Similarly, massage of the neck and whole back, following a downward movement from the neck along the spine, may also relieve tension in that area.

During treatment the masseur will look for indications about the patient, such as the distribution of muscular tension throughout the body. Such information is invaluable to the physician, allowing a deeper insight into the causes of the condition and other interrelated, underlying disorders.

Depending on the patient's condition, the doctor may prescribe a

remedy to counterbalance the symptom which is based on the allopathic principle or he/she may use a remedy based on the homoeopathic principle of matching the remedy to an illness. He/she may even consider a combination of substances that will work on the illness in different complementary ways. Migraine is a good example of this.

Anthroposophical doctors believe that migraine is caused by the blood vessels of the brain at first narrowing in spasm and then becoming dilated, with a seeping of fluid in the surrounding tissue. In anthroposophical parlance, 'the problem involves a blood process (related to the metabolic system) in the brain (nerve–sense system). The initial symptom is a contraction and tightening (characteristic of the nerve–sense system), followed by an excessive dilation of the blood vessels (metabolic system)' (*Anthroposophical Medicine* by Evans and Rodger, page 79).

As migraine is considered to result from the predominance of the metabolic processes in the head, which is the centre of the nerve–sense system, the therapeutic aim is to reduce the metabolic activity in that area. Therefore an anthroposophical preparation called Bidor (trade name) is often used for headaches and particularly for migraine. It contains quartz and sulphur combined with iron (ferrous sulphate and silica). Primarily, Bidor's action is aimed at harmonising the fundamental imbalance of the nervous and metabolic systems, which is at the root of the headache. It is not a painkiller. It means, therefore, that Bidor can be used for prevention as well as for alleviating the symptoms and comes in different strengths – e.g. 1% for a course of treatment to lessen frequency and severity of attacks or 5% when an attack is coming on.

A Conversation With An Anthroposophical Doctor

Q: Where do you place headaches and migraines in the anthroposophical system of medicine?
A: An anthroposophical physician will try to identify the imbalance in the relationships of the three organ systems. Migraines and headaches are very common symptoms of such an imbalance.

The central nervous system orders and regulates the metabolic activity

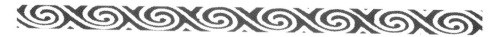

in the body. If the sense–nerve system is weakened, the 'inflammatory frenzy' of the metabolic process can take over and predominate. The sense–nerve system would be overwhelmed by excess metabolic activity. The symptoms that result in this situation are: impaired thought and concentration, throbbing pain, flashing lights, nausea and vomiting. The patient has to lie still, in a darkened room. Light, sound, movement and touch is painful. Breathing is shallow.

Our cool and clear head is (metabolically) 'on fire'.

Q: Food allergies are now thought to be the main cause of migraine. What is the anthroposophical medical view on this?
A: In our view, the sense–nerve system is weakened in its task to regulate and control the metabolic activity. In that case, foodstuffs cannot be properly integrated and the body can have a hypersensitive (allergic) reaction to them, leading to migraine, as described above. Essentially, our view is that migraine is caused by the underlying weak relationship between the nerve–sense system and the metabolic system.

Q: I understand that massage is considered by anthroposophical practitioners to be particularly therapeutic for tension headaches. If so, why?
A: Massage is an invaluable therapy for the rapid relief of tension headache, as well as part of a long-term treatment for recurring migraine. So often, ingrained muscular tension patterns have established themselves and equally disturbed patterns of warmth-distribution (cold feet and hands). Through rhythmical organisation in this way, the balance between the three systems can be restored.

Q: Are there specific medications or therapies that you would recommend for common headaches or migraines?
A: The preparation Bidor was mentioned earlier. This is a standard (or typical) remedy, that is used for all types of headaches. It contains three substances that are almost archetypal for the three systems; Silica (clarity of the head), Sulphur (representing the metabolic) and Iron (mediating between the two). Additionally, a careful individual assessment can lead to other, more specifically tailored medicines and treatment.

Often a course of eurythmy is very helpful, again to support and strengthen the rhythmic system. Therapeutic painting can also be very effective. Dietary advice and life-style should be looked at. The point is that a therapeutic 'composition', or regime, is planned out of the range of possibilities available.

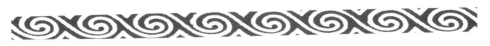

Finding A Practitioner

Anthroposophical practitioners are all qualified medical doctors who have taken a further postgraduate course recognised by the Anthroposophical Medical Association in Britain. Some may be found working in the NHS, although others work privately or in the Rudolf Steiner schools and homes for children. Residential treatment in certain private clinics is also available.

Consultations are very much like seeing a GP except that there may be additional details and questions about, for example, lifestyle and emotional conditions. Diagnosis is made in the same way as a GP and treatment is prescribed depending on the individual characteristics of the patient.

Treatment may be by conventional, anthroposophical, herbal or homoeopathic remedies. Practitioners may try and bring about long-term changes, in addition to alleviating symptoms, by prescribing eurhythmy or an art therapy in order to sort out an underlying imbalance, and might send a patient to a specialist.

The Anthroposophical Medical Association maintains a register of members. It is based at the Park Attwood Therapeutic Centre, Trimpley, Bewdley, Worcestershire DY12 1RE.

Further Reading

Anthroposophical Medicine by Dr M Evans and I Rodger (Thorsons)
Anthroposophical Medicine and its Remedies by Otto Wolf (Weleda Ag)
Rudolf Steiner: Scientist of the Invisible by A P Shepherd (Floris Books)

7

ACUPUNCTURE AND ACUPRESSURE

In Chinese philosophy all living matter is activated by a life force or energy called *chi*. It is claimed that in the human body this energy flows along channels called *meridians*. As long as the *chi* flows freely, optimum health is maintained.

Traditional Chinese medicine views the state of ill-health as the result of an impairment or imbalance in the free flow of *chi*. This occurs when two opposite but complementary parts – a *yin* aspect and a *yang* aspect – are not balanced. (*Yin* is understood to express cold, wetness and darkness, while *yang* has the qualities of heat, brightness and dryness.)

Treatment concentrates on restoring this lost equilibrium. One of the best-known methods is acupuncture in which the body's energy network is entered by inserting needles to stimulate specific points to restore the *yin/yang* equilibrium. Another technique is to stimulate the points by way of finger pressure and massage. This is called acupressure.

Acupuncture's success in treating certain diseases is now accepted and it has grown in popularity over the last few decades in the West, even if exactly how it works is open to controversy and further research.

The needles used are very fine and puncture the skin at defined points along the body to stimulate the flow of *chi* energy and to remove any blockages. There are about 800 acupuncture points. These points join up to form 12 major meridians that, apart from the *triple warmer*, are named after the organs to which they relate, namely, the *large intestine, stomach, heart, spleen, small intestine, bladder, circulation, kidney, gall-bladder, lung* and *liver*. In addition, there are two other central and governing meridians.

Origins Of Acupuncture

The origins of the theory of *chi* lie in ancient China although it is unclear how acupuncture was discovered. It is claimed that about

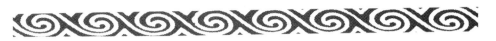

4,000 years ago it was observed that warriors who were wounded by arrows miraculously recovered from diseases that had been troubling them for many years. It was also noticed that certain organs seemed to be associated with specific points on the body which often became tender when the body was diseased and that these points could be used for the treatment of disorders.

The original needles were made from stone and did not penetrate the skin; bone and bamboo needles did, but these were used later. Undoubtedly, a cause-and-effect relationship was worked out by noting the point punctured and the disease it cured. When metal was discovered, the needles were made from copper, silver, gold and other alloys.

The earliest written record dates from the time of the Yellow Emperor Huang Ti, who lived in the Warring States period in China (475–221 BC), and has been reprinted in modern times as the *Yellow Emperor's Classic of Internal Medicine.*

Acupuncture was introduced to the West during the Ching dynasty (1644–1911) although the Chinese themselves attempted to ban it for political reasons. It reached Germany in the seventeenth century and then France in the middle of the nineteenth century. Due to pressure from the Western powers, which effectively ruled China at this time, the Chinese government again tried to ban traditional medicine in 1922, but its practice continued covertly until it was positively espoused by Chairman Mao in the aftermath of the Second World War when acupuncture treatment and research was given fresh impetus and energy.

Even today acupuncture has great grass-roots support. In China, especially, the motivation behind the promotion of acupuncture has been the relative poverty of the country and the lack of 'conventionally' trained physicians, drugs and medical equipment – but also because it works well in primary health-care situations. Indeed, acupuncture is used widely by the general population and needles and other equipment can be purchased in shops as easily as aspirin can be bought in the West.

The West's interest in acupuncture was initially fuelled by the writings of the French diplomat Soulie de Morant in the 1940s. Later, acupuncture was brought to the attention of the West during the presidency of Richard Nixon. While visiting Peking, to report on 'ping-pong diplomacy' the renowned American commentator James Reston contracted acute appendicitis which required immediate surgery. This was successfully carried out under local anaesthetic

while the postoperative pain was treated with acupuncture. This so impressed him that he visited many other centres where acupuncture was practised and, on his return to the USA, he did much to focus both professional and public attention on this therapy.

How And Why Does Acupuncture Work?

The fact is, Western scientific approaches to medicine cannot explain how acupuncture works. One theory is that acupuncture encourages the body to release natural painkillers, such as *endorphins,* and *enkephalins,* which are known to be especially beneficial for cases of depression and allergies. The painkilling effect of acupuncture is also attributed to the 'gate control' theory that there are *neuropathway gates* to the brain via the spinal chord. Anaesthetic acupuncture is believed to close the gates, blocking the pain messages so that we do not feel the pain. While this may account for the anaesthetic effects, it does not explain why acupuncture can heal non-painful conditions.

Some sceptics attribute the success of acupuncture to the placebo effect – that the patient, just by believing that it works, stimulates the body's own healing mechanisms, but this does not explain the long tradition of veterinary acupuncture. Or they say dismissively that it is 'mind over matter'. Some people compare acupuncture to the power of suggestion associated with hypnosis, with its state of heightened awareness which stimulates physiological changes. Again, it is difficult to establish how acupuncture works, but it is certainly very effective.

Diagnosis

In order to diagnose a patient's condition, the acupuncturist will take a full medical history and observe particular features, such as the appearance of the face, tongue (in itself a highly refined diagnostic tool) and eyes, and the condition of the skin. Aspects such as the distinctive odour of the body, personal gestures and voice tone will assist the practitioner in making a diagnosis. However, practitioners vary their approach, and some also make a physical examination or include medical tests.

The next procedure is to check the pulses, of which there are 12, one for each meridian, six to each wrist. There are 28 qualities that

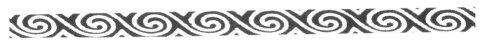

can be recognised from the pulses, including *tight, hasty, thin, weak, fine* and *slow*. This technique, which takes years to master, gives the acupuncturist an insight into the gravity of the disorder and how to treat it. Pulse diagnosis is one of the main methods of determining the condition of body-energy flow.

On completion of the diagnosis, the acupuncturist decides which acupuncture points to manipulate in order to restore the balance in the patient's energy pattern. Each point has a particular function attributed to it and it is according to this that the practitioner decides which points are to be stimulated.

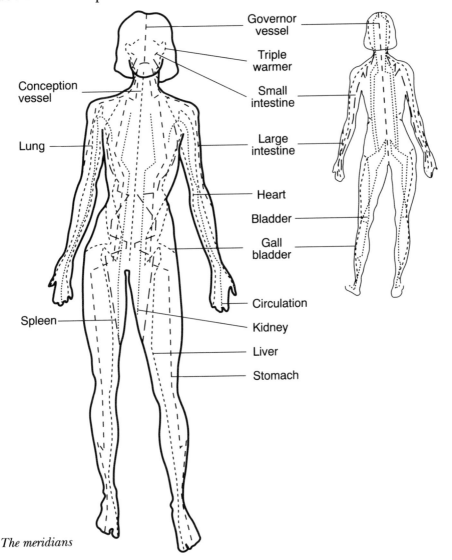

Governor vessel

Triple warmer

Conception vessel

Small intestine

Lung

Large intestine

Heart

Bladder

Gall bladder

Circulation

Spleen

Kidney

Liver

Stomach

The meridians

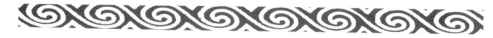

The Use Of Needles

The first reaction to the use of needles is usually revulsion, or fear at the thought of the pain that might be felt when they are inserted. Memories of painful injections or pinpricks are revived. But, according to those who undergo acupuncture, it is a relatively painless procedure. Insertion by a skilled practitioner feels a bit like a small pinprick followed by a sensation of tingling, fullness or pressure. When performed correctly, it draws no blood and the sensation lasts only a short time afterwards.

The very fine needles are inserted obliquely, vertically or almost horizontally, usually only a fraction of an inch into the skin, although there are many other kinds of needle if specialised treatment is needed. Deeper insertion may be required but this is not felt to be any more painful than lighter insertion.

For some acupuncture treatments a ball of dried mugwort or wormwood herb may be placed on the top of the needle's handle and set alight. A gentle heat is produced which conducts down through the needle and increases the effectiveness of the stimulation. This form of treatment is known as *moxibustion.*

Some practitioners use electrical techniques whereby a device is used to produce an alternating electrical current which is passed down the needle into the skin. Other electrical instruments may be used to detect the points which need to be stimulated, as it is known that acupuncture points are associated with decreased electrical resistance and so can be identified in this way. Electro-acupuncture is not common but may be available, depending on the practitioner. It is claimed to regulate the required energy flow with more precision and this is mostly used for analgesia.

Another form of acupuncture, known as *auriculotherapy,* relies solely on the ear. It is based on the correlation between the ear and other parts of the body, the ear resembling the position of the human foetus in the womb (inverted with the head pointing downwards). Two hundred points on the ear have been found for treatment. This is usually carried out by an electronic instrument that detects the points and simultaneously stimulates them, although needles are often used. In China, small seeds are placed on points with a sticking plaster and the patient then applies pressure on the seed several times a day.

Pain Relief For Headaches And Migraine

Acupuncture is commonly used to alleviate pain and in China is sometimes the only anaesthetic resorted to. Relief for chronic pain can be effected without the side-effects of drugs. The success of the technique depends, however, on the nature of the problem and how far advanced it is.

Headaches can often be due to an energy blockage in the *yang* channel in the head. The location of the pain and the correct diagnosis will determine the points used.

Acupressure

When you hold your forehead or press your temples during a headache or rub your palms briskly in cold weather, you are instinctively practising the ancient Chinese art of acupressure. More than 5,000 years ago, the Chinese discovered that by applying pressure to certain points on the body they were able to gain relief from symptoms of pain.

Acupressure uses the fingers to press certain points on the body to stimulate its healing powers. When these points just under the surface of the skin are pressed they release muscular tension and promote the circulation of blood. This healing can relieve stress, enable the body to relax and generally promote a sense of well-being.

The points used are the same as those in acupuncture. While acupuncture has had greater recognition, due to the amount of scientific research carried out on it, acupressure, the older of the two traditions, is an increasingly popular self-treatment therapy for tension-related conditions. It requires no instruments (all you need are your fingers), no potions or tablets, has no side-effects and can be practised anywhere.

Headaches, arthritis, backache, muscle ache, insomnia and tension caused by stress can all be helped by the correct use of acupressure points. It is not too difficult to learn the simple techniques and they can be practised on oneself or others quite safely if one follows the guidelines properly. The effect is much enhanced by using the method of trigger point stimulation in combination with breathing exercises and relaxation techniques.

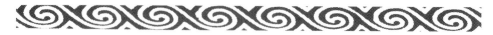

How It Works

Called *potent points*, acupressure points are believed to be sensitive to bioelectrical impulses in the body. The Chinese consider them to be junctions of the special pathways through which *chi* passes.

Acupressure can help to dissolve the tension which concentrates around these points. Fatigue and stress cause muscle fibres to contract, due to the secretion of lactic acid. Pressing the points enables the muscle fibres to elongate which improves the blood circulation and enables the body to remove toxins. This aids the immune system and therefore increases the body's resistance to illness.

Definition Of Points

- *Local point:* this is a point which is in the same area as the pain or tension. Relief is felt when this point is stimulated. In China, these points are known as *ashi* points, literally meaning 'That's it!'
- *Trigger point:* when the local point is stimulated, it can relieve pain in a distant area. This triggering mechanism is thought to work because the stimulus is conveyed through the meridians
- *Tonic point:* these are specific points in the body that maintain general health. A popular tonic point is in the webbing between the thumb and the index finger.

Locating The Points

The name of each point offers an insight into its use. For example, the *Three Mile Point* is supposed to give a person energy equivalent to that required to run three miles! This point has been used effectively by athletes to increase stamina and endurance.

Each point has also been assigned a number and this system is universally used by practitioners of acupuncture and acupressure. The points can be located by reference to anatomical pointers, such as bone indentations and other organs. Some points lie in a knot in a muscle and the skill of the practitioner lies in correctly locating the points. This is important for the specific management of certain conditions. However, as stated before, acupressure can be practised for the self-treatment of many minor ailments.

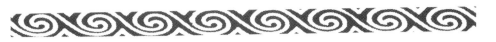

The Practice Of Acupressure

There are several different ways of practising acupressure. The basic technique is to use thumbs, fingers, palms or the backs of the hand to apply firm pressure on a point for a specified period of time. To relieve pain, apply gradual pressure and hold without any movement for a few minutes. A minute or so of steady pressure will calm and relax the nervous system.

Kneading the muscles as you would knead dough can make muscles more pliable and soft. This is usually used for the calf muscle. On tender areas, such as the face, tapping with the fingers will improve the functioning of the nerves. Brisk rubbing will stimulate the lymphatic system and generally increase circulation.

Potent Points For Headaches And Migraine

Headaches are not just considered as expressions of a physical ailment but are also connected with the emotional and spiritual aspects of a person.

- Called the *Gates of Consciousness*, these points are to be found just below the base of the skull in the hollow between the two vertical neck muscles. Use your thumbs to press the points for 2 minutes, slowly tilting your head back while maintaining pressure. This point is particularly beneficial for migraine.
- Located in a hollow in the centre of the back of the head under the base of the skull, this point is called *Wind Mansion*. Press this point using your right thumb, at the same time as pressing *Drilling Bamboo*, located in the upper hollow of the eye socket near the bridge of the nose, with your index finger and left thumb. Tilt back your head and breathe deeply for 2 minutes.
- Called *Facial Beauty*, these points are located at the bottom of the cheekbones below the centre of your eyes. Using your middle and index fingers apply gentle pressure upwards for a minute or so. This is particularly recommended for congestion headaches.
- The point called *Joining the Valley* lies between the thumb and the index finger. Place your right hand on top of your left hand and press the webbing between the thumb and index finger towards the bone that connects with the index finger. This should be done for a minute. Repeat for the right hand. This is especially beneficial for frontal headaches. (***Caution:* pregnant women should not use this point because it can cause premature contraction of the uterus.**)

Acupressure points

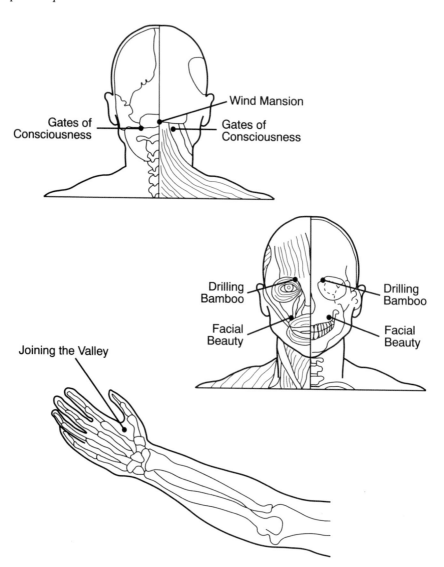

Acupressure Massage

There are several massage techniques and each therapist may have his/her own way of working. Practitioners will usually use a firm thumb or the fingertips to massage the pain relieving points, although some may use palms, elbows and even knees.

The sessions typically last between 30 and 60 minutes. Depending on your condition, they may be needed for several weeks or longer.

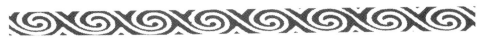

For tension headaches, pain relief may be rapid, but long-standing conditions, such as migraine, would require a course of treatment in conjunction with dietary measures and other complementary healing techniques.

As the nature of this therapy lends itself to administration at home you can practise acupressure on yourself, or ask a relative or friend to do it for you. It would, however, be advisable first to follow a course in the technique by a practitioner.

Finding A Practitioner

The fact that anyone can call themselves an acupuncturist makes it all the more important that you establish that the practitioner is properly trained. There are four professional bodies which are affiliated to the Council for Acupuncture, 38 Mount Pleasant, London WC1X OAP, which maintains a register of practitioners. They are the British Acupuncture Association and Register, the International Register of Oriental Medicine UK, the Register of Traditional Chinese Medicine, and the Traditional Medicine Society. Before qualifying, students have to undergo a minimum 3-year course which includes such subjects as anatomy, diagnosis, pathology and physiology.

Further Reading

Acupressure: Headway Lifeguides by Eliana Harvey & Mary Jane Oatley (Headway) publishing late 1994
Acupressure's Potent Points by Michael Reed Gach (Bantam Books)
Acupuncture by Alexander Macdonald (George Allen & Unwin)
The Acupuncture Treatment of Pain by Leon Chaitow (Thorsons)

8

AROMATHERAPY: MORE THAN JUST AROMATIC ASPIRIN

Aromatherapy uses plant essences to treat various disorders. The Bible records the use of plants and their oils for similar purposes and the Egyptians used aromatic oils widely, for medicines and embalming as well as perfumes. On opening the tomb of Tutankhamun, scientists were amazed to discover that a faint smell of aromatic oils from the embalmed corpse was still perceptible. The Romans also used plant essences for cookery and medicine and it was they who introduced the use of essential oils into the British Isles. The earliest written text, however, is Chinese and dates back to 1000–700 BC.

The Middle Ages in Europe saw a decline in the study of medicine, but in the cultures of the Chinese, Indian and Arab peoples it flourished and advanced. Amid their many discoveries was the invention of the process of steam distillation, particularly significant to aromatherapy as it made the extraction of the essential oil from the plant a viable proposition. This is credited to the Arab physician and philosopher Abu Ibn Sina, known in the West as Avicenna, and his technique is still in use, relatively unchanged, today.

The Renaissance saw the rebirth of European culture and the study and development of medicine similarly flowered. Colonial exploration and the opening up of the Americas enabled a number of new plant species to be introduced into Europe. Subsequent centuries saw an increase in the extraction and use of essential plant oils for antiseptics, perfumes and medicines.

Once chemistry began to flourish, especially during the nineteenth century, chemical copies of essential oils were produced, as they were cheap and relatively easy to manufacture. But they were ineffective as treatments and tended to be used mainly for perfumes. Even when scientists managed to produce the synthetic properties of the oils, they did not have the same therapeutic effect

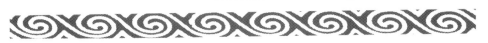

and the use of essential oils declined.

The present century has witnessed the re-emergence of interest in aromatherapy. This can be ascribed to the French doctor René Gattefosse who accidentally discovered the healing power of the essential oils. He burned his hand and immediately plunged it into the nearest liquid, which happened to be lavender oil. On seeing how quickly the burned hand healed, leaving no scarring, he went on to investigate the properties and effects of other essential oils and used many to treat wounded soldiers in the First World War. It was through the writings of Gattefosse that the actual word 'aromatherapy' was coined. After Gattefosse's death there were many people who carried on his work. Prominent among them was the French physician Jean Valnet who used essential oils of clove, lemon and chamomile as natural disinfectants and antiseptics to fumigate hospital wards and to sterilise surgical instruments. The link between aromatherapy and the cosmetic industry was forged and developed by a French biochemist, Marguerite Maury, who was instrumental in developing the aromatherapeutic massage techniques.

How Aromatherapy Works

Aromatherapy is holistic – influencing the mind, body and spirit. Whereas the mind/body connection is perhaps more appreciable and can be explained, the spiritual aspect is much more elusive, as is the case with many holistic therapies.

Different odours are said to stimulate the brain and to evoke images or feelings associated with that particular smell. While this process is not yet fully understood, it is thought that because the area of the brain associated with smell is closely connected with the *limbic* area of the brain (the part concerned with emotion, memory and intuition), aromatherapy can be used to influence mind and body. Different smells are used to relax or to stimulate, depending on the requirements of the patient. It is widely recognised that our sense of smell can engender changes in emotional behaviour. Indeed, the olfactory nerves, which are the nerves concerned with the sense of smell, affect memory and thinking, and so different odours evoke images or feelings that are associated with them.

Touching is also essential for good health. In our early lives as babies and young children it is the most important medium through which love is communicated. The use of massage in aromatherapy

builds on this. The pleasurable sensation of being touched induces feelings of being loved and cared for. Combining massage with essential oils is central to the practice of aromatherapy, both for general relaxation and for the treatment of specific problem areas.

Using Essential Oils

Essential oils are considered by many to be the 'life force' of a plant, exercising almost mystical powers. They are found in all plants and herbs, giving fragrance or flavour. They are extracted from all parts of the plant, from leaves and flowers, roots, seeds and rinds.

There are various extraction techniques. The most common is steam distillation where steam is passed under pressure through the plant material. The heat causes the release and evaporation of the oil which then passes through a water cooler where it condenses and is collected. Solvent extractions in which the flowers are covered with a solvent, such as petrol ether, is sometimes used to extract the oil. When the solvent evaporates the oil is left behind. Some oils, mainly from citrus fruits, may be extracted through expression. This involves the rinds being pressed or grated. The oils from the torn cells are collected in a sponge and squeezed out.

The average yield of essential oil from a plant substance is 1.5%, which means that about 70 kg of plant material will make just 1 kg of essential oil. Of course, yields vary, depending on the nature of the plant, the time it is harvested and the quality of the soil it is grown in. Jasmine harvested at sunset will yield the greatest amount of oil, while rose has so little that it may take 100 kg of some varieties of rose petals to make half a litre of oil. The final price of the essential oil depends on yield, which is why rose is the most expensive of the essential oils.

How the essential oils actually work is not entirely clear but they are believed to promote a state of well-being and harmony in the mind, apart from the oil's particular therapeutic properties. They all share the properties of being powerful antiseptics which destroy bacteria and viruses. They stimulate the immune system, thereby encouraging the body to resist disease, as well as alleviating pain and reducing fluid retention.

Chemically complex substances themselves, essential oils have a similarly complicated effect on the body. They may contain up to a hundred chemical components in varying amounts and each constituent, however minor, may perform some vital function. This

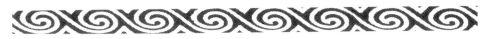

is why synthetic equivalents are unlikely to equal in performance the natural essential oils. For example, when the major constituent of lemongrass oil, an *aldehyde citral,* was extracted and chemically synthesised it produced an allergic reaction when applied to the skin. However, lemongrass oil itself does not produce an allergic reaction. Testing has shown that the other minor constituents in naturally produced lemongrass oil help to neutralise the harmful effects of the aldehyde citral.

How essential oils act upon the body may partly be explained by considering the way in which they are absorbed into the bloodstream. Essential oils pass into the skin and then diffuse into the *capillaries* (extremely narrow blood vessels) from where they enter the main bloodstream to exercise their therapeutic effects on the body. Aromatic massage, baths or neat applications of essential oils therefore, all form a part of therapeutic treatment.

The aromatic molecules of essential oils can also be absorbed via the lungs, from where they diffuse across the air sacs into the surrounding capillaries and then into the main blood vessels. This is how aromatic inhalation works.

Smell And Touch

It is widely recognised that our sense of smell works on a subconscious level and this, in turn, means that smell can engender changes in emotional behaviour. Indeed, the *olfactory nerves,* which are concerned with the sense of smell, affect memory and thought, and different odours may evoke images or feelings that are associated with a particular aroma or odour. This is possibly how aromatherapy deals with the emotional and mental aspects of healing. Different smells may be used to relax or stimulate, depending on the needs of the patient.

Touching is essential for health. Indeed, mothers of newborn babies are encouraged to touch and hold their babies frequently so as to communicate love and well-being. Massage similarly induces the feeling of being loved and cared for and is beneficial at any age.

There are physical benefits, too. The action of massage stimulates the immune system, reduces high blood pressure and improves the circulation of the blood and lymph system. It also reduces muscular tension or swelling, as well as relieving pain in the muscles and joints. Its main effect is to aid relaxation, which is vital for the healing process. Relaxation alleviates psychological tension and helps to soothe turbulent emotions.

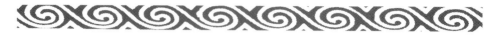

Combining massage with essential oils is the central practice of aromatherapy, both for general relaxation and for the treatment of specific problem areas. Some major organs of the body, such as the large intestine, are accessible to massage, while more internally placed organs, such as the liver and kidneys, may be treated by massaging the area of the body where they are situated. This is believed to stimulate the ailing organs by increasing the local blood supply and galvanising the nerves. Aromatherapists sometimes use the pressure point techniques found in acupressure and reflexology, as using massage with essential oils on the relevant pressure points stimulates specific internal organs.

In Baths

Used in baths, essential oils may act either as tonics or sedatives. Hot water opens pores and helps the body to absorb the oils more quickly. Bathing with essential oils added to the water also relieves the effects of stress and alleviates muscular pain.

Aromatherapy And Stress

Many illnesses are at least partially caused by stress and among them are stress-related headaches. Although stress is common in our daily lives, it becomes a serious problem when a person is no longer able to cope with it. This may in turn engender a serious illness. Aromatherapy, which emphasises the importance of dealing with stress, can be seen as a preventive type of therapy. Dealing with stress in its early stages may forestall a more dangerous illness.

Massage will confer upon the recipient feelings of peace and relaxation, providing time to think and perhaps to put a more realistic perspective upon any problems. Pent-up emotions may be released.

The combination of massage and essential oils is particularly effective. The essential oils work on the mental tension while massage alleviates the physical tension. Indeed, the effects of an aromatic massage often include dramatic improvements in sleeping patterns, leading to heightened vitality and physical energy. So stress-related disorders, such as digestive problems, headaches, acne and other skin conditions, may be treated effectively by aromatherapy. This is partly due to the release of mood-inducing chemicals in the brain and body which act as stimulants and sedatives.

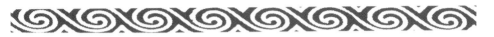

Some essential oils cause the release of natural painkillers, thereby relieving the distress caused by bee and wasp stings, toothaches and headaches.

Headaches And Migraine

Headaches

- Stress-related headaches may be relieved by a head massage with aromatic oils, concentrating on the back of the neck, on the temples and around the eyes. Useful essential oils include basil, chamomile, lavender, marjoram, rosemary and peppermint.
- Compresses on the eyes using chamomile, rosemary and parsley are soothing.
- For congestive headaches where there is catarrh build-up, inhalation is best. Once the catarrh is removed from the sinuses, the headaches will go. Useful oils are cajeput, geranium, neroli and tea tree oils.
- For a hangover headache, a long, hot bath with pepper and juniper clears the head.
- Sniffing from a bottle of peppermint may relieve some headaches.

Migraines

- Oils for migraine include chamomile, fennel, lemongrass, marjoram, melissa and oregano – massage the temples and neck.
- Peppermint is helpful for a migraine accompanied by stomach pain.
- Congestion-related migraines can be helped by basil or eucalyptus, and nausea relieved by aniseed, chamomile or lavender.

Treatment

Headaches and migraines can be successfully treated at home, using essential oils. Keeping aromatic oils handy for burns, stings or headaches or perhaps, to put in a bath, is a sensible alternative to orthodox treatment for such common minor ailments.

When purchasing oils for self-administration, you should ensure that they come from a reliable source. In particular, you should only purchase oils that come in tightly sealed dark glass bottles – oils are damaged by ultraviolet light and those sold in clear plastic bottles in some high street stores have little aromatherapeutic value. At home they should also be kept stored in dark glass bottles (green, brown

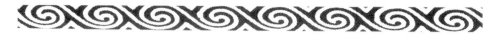

or blue) in cool conditions, although not in the refrigerator.

Oils should be handled with care, as some can be potentially dangerous in the hands of an inexperienced user. So for a serious condition or a long-term disorder, a visit to an aromatherapist is to be recommended. In any event, it is difficult to lie down and massage oneself properly, even if the right blend and mixture of essential oils has been selected. This is even more difficult when you are feeling ill.

A consultation with an aromatherapist begins with a discussion in which the therapist enquires not only about the nature of the problem but also about general health and lifestyle. Diet, exercise, appearance and sleeping habits are all relevant. Foot reflexology may be incorporated to determine more about the ailment.

The nature of the problem determines whether the therapist prescribes massage, inhalation or another technique. He/she will mix oils that suit your condition and which appeal aesthetically to you. Treatment usually consists of six sessions, although more may be needed on an *ad hoc* or long-term basis, particularly for migraines.

Finding An Aromatherapist

For a list of practitioners or further information write, sending a SAE to:

International Federation of Aromatherapists, Department of Continuing Education, Royal Masonic Hospital, Ravenscourt Park, London W6 OTN;

Aromatherapy Organisations Council, 3 Latymer Close, Braybrooke, Market Harborough, Leicestershire LE16 8LN.

Further Reading

Aromatherapy: Headway Lifeguides by Denise Brown (Headway)
Aromatherapy by Daniele Ryman (Piatkus)
Aromatherapy: A Definitive Guide To Essential Oils by Lisa Chidell (Headway)
Aromatherapy – Massage With Essential Oils by Christine Wildwood (Element Books)
Massage: Headway Lifeguides by Denise Brown (Headway)
The Art of Aromatherapy by Robert Tisserand (C W Daniel)

REFLEXOLOGY: PAIN RELIEF FROM TOE TO HEAD

Reflexology is a method whereby 'reflex areas' of the foot are massaged in order to affect areas in the body that are at a distance from the part treated on the foot, but are connected to it. It is derived from an ancient form of Chinese medicine and its basic principles have been used throughout the ages.

The technique dates back at least 5,000 years. Traditional Chinese medicine has always applied massage to the feet, hands and body to affect internal organs and muscles. The ancient Egyptians must also have used reflexology techniques, if the drawings on tombs, which depict feet being held and massaged, are anything to go by. Some native American tribes, and tribal populations in Africa, use a form of reflexology as part of their medicine.

Modern reflexology owes much to 'zone therapy', practised by the American physician Dr William Fitzgerald. He was intrigued by his observation that with some of his patients he was able to carry out operations on the throat and nose without their being in any significant pain, yet on others, the same sort of operation caused a great deal of pain. He began his investigations in 1913 and found that in those cases where there had been little pain the patient had been applying pressure to parts of the hand. In other cases, prior to the operation he had applied pressure to certain areas of the body, and this was subsequently found to inhibit pain in other areas. In fact, we often use this technique in our daily lives without realising what we are doing. For example, as an automatic response to pain, we may bite or grind our teeth or, perhaps, rub our hands in an effort to lessen the hurt we are experiencing elsewhere in our bodies.

Dr Fitzgerald went on to practise a technique which he called 'zone therapy'. He divided the body up into ten longitudinal zones, from the head downwards to both toes and fingers. He believed that the body's bioelectrical energy flowed down these pathways to reflex points in the hands and feet.

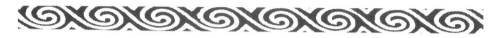

These initial findings were tentatively received by the medical profession, although a few doctors were prepared to give them serious analysis. Dr Joe Riley investigated the claims and a protegée of his, Eunice Ingham, pioneered the 'Ingham Compression Method of Reflexology,' concentrating on sensitive areas on the feet, and encouraged massage to the toes as well as the soles and tops of the feet. The introduction of reflexology into Britain was largely through the efforts of Mrs Doreen Bayley, herself influenced by Eunice Ingham.

So reflexology has developed from the general principles of zone therapy, where certain points on the feet influence other parts of the body which are seemingly unconnected.

Of late, a link between reflexology and acupuncture has been suggested.

The Role Of The Feet

Reflexologists consider that the whole body is represented in the shape and contours of the feet and that a map of the body could be drawn on the soles of the feet. The right foot represents the right side of the body and the left foot the left side. Terminal endings, or *pressure points*, are found mainly in the soles, but energy channels (*meridians*) can be stimulated or pressured at the sides and on the tops of the feet and also up the sides of the ankles, where the meridians enter or leave.

An imaginary line drawn across each foot, halfway down, corresponds to the waistline of the body. The big toes represent the head, neck and their structures. Facial sinuses are to be found on the other toes, whilst eye and ear structures are located at the roots of the smaller four toes. Areas below the body waistline will be located in regions of the feet closer to the heels.

The basis of treatment is the belief that the body's energy flows through energy channels, referred to as *meridians*. The energy is the life force or vital energy flow. Meridians arise from all organs and structures in the body, joining larger meridians at various energy centres. Five major channels on either side of the midline collect all the flows, accumulating all sources before reaching the periphery in the hands and feet. The energy flows return inwards from the periphery, back to their sources, much like the circulatory system.

Acupuncturists insert needles to intercept these energy flows at specific points all around the body. Acupressure can also be used at

these points to elicit pain relief and treatment before or beyond the point of pressure or interception. But reflexologists locate their treatments to the hands and feet of clients, especially to the feet, which give the best response. Due to gravity, sediments accumulate in the periphery (the furthest points prior to return) and these are felt as granules under the skin. With the whole life force gravitating to concentrated areas of hands and feet, access to the client's energy flows is afforded.

A reflexologist sees the body as a whole, as an energy flow that may be impeded. Any blockage along the flow means that structures beyond the blockage are not at maximum efficiency and, if they are not already in disorder they will surely and eventually succumb to problems. Treatment is always of the whole, since the whole affects the part, and vice versa.

A reflexologist will spend time at a troubled pressure point in the foot, not only to treat the blocked area and its locating structures, but mainly to harmonise or balance the whole of the flow. If we are imbalanced, we are not at our best potential.

Reflexes on both feet

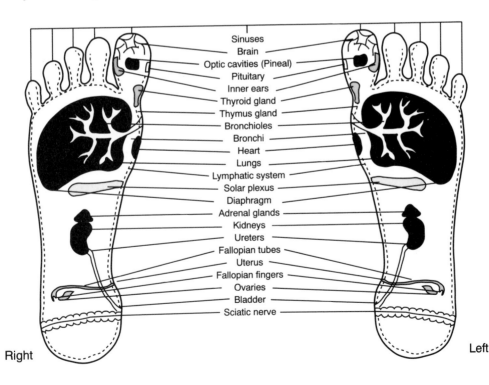

Right   Left

How it works

It is thought that a number of changes take place in the body during a reflexology treatment. One change is an extra production of edomorphines, substances that act as the body's own natural pain relievers. Edomorphines are at least five times more powerful than morphine.

The pituitary gland is triggered to release messenger endomorphines, when pain arises in the body. These cause pain-blocking endomorphines to be released near the sites of pains to inhibit pain signals passing into the central nervous system, through the spinal cord. But if pain is severe or multiple, the system becomes overloaded and its function less effective and pain is not relieved. At this time, sufferers use analgesics or seek professional help. Analgesics generally mask the pain but do not correct the problem.

Uses Of Reflexology

Reflexology is useful for simple acute conditions such as colds, and for functional problems such as constipation. For serious long-term diseases it can be helpful but will take longer. It can help relieve conditions such as asthma, headaches and migraines (more details later) and other stress-related problems, because it also aids relaxation. Emergencies would be better treated by other therapeutic systems.

Reflexologists do not diagnose disorders, only discuss areas of possibilities. If there is a problem in a specific area its corresponding reflex point in the foot, when massaged, should register pain or show evidence of blockage through toxic build-up. However, experience indicates that there may be a disorder in the corresponding organ, not what the problem is or its gravity.

Reflexology is probably most beneficial as part of an integrated treatment, rather than being regarded as a therapy that can cure, although it may help effect one. It acts to encourage the body to heal itself by restoring energy imbalances and bodily workings. Therefore it may be seen more as a preventive therapy which is able to forestall the development of a more serious disorder by encouraging good health and proper bodily processes. Many reflexologists claim that, through reflexology, early warning signs of potential problems can be picked up and treated.

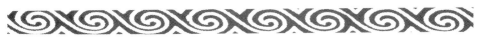

Visiting A Therapist

Self-help is possible for simple conditions, although a visit to a therapist first may help you to apply the techniques yourself later on. For a serious disorder or for a specific problem, visiting a reflexologist is usually necessary.

The therapist is likely to counsel you about diet, stress levels and lifestyle, and will discuss your medical history, sensitively and in confidence. Your awareness and co-operation will greatly improve your response to treatment.

The sessions will commence with an all-round foot massage during which the therapist will go over the feet applying acupressure massage to the points and encouraging you to comment as to whether any pain is felt. As a first step, the therapist will attempt to relax you by releasing tension from the ankles and feet. With general massage, one technique is to gently rotate the right foot from the ankle joint, followed by a rotation of the toes. Simple massage and movements will help to relax the foot and hence the patient. Crystal deposits will be taken as a sign of energy blockage and, after the general all-over foot massage, the therapist will concentrate on the problem areas. Sessions usually last for an hour and a treatment programme usually consists of six to eight sessions with further top-up sessions at longer intervals if necessary. You may find that your body starts to display signs of detoxification. These may be, for example, a cold, aching joints, sore throats or diarrhoea. These are not a cause for alarm but are, rather, to be welcomed. They mean that the therapy is working. In any event, they will not last for long.

Headaches And Migraine

Depending on the cause of the headache and migraine the corresponding pressure points will be treated. The reflex points to the head are found on all the toes including the big toe. Other associated reflex areas are also treated. These usually include the neck, cervical spine, sinuses, eyes, solar plexus, intestines, stomach, liver and gall-bladder. For women experiencing headaches or migraine because of hormonal changes or which are related to the menstrual cycle, the reflex areas relating to the reproductive organs are also massaged.

If you are going to administer reflexology on a self-help basis, it is recommended that you attend a proper teaching seminar as it is

important to know just where the zones are located on the feet and the specific massage techniques that are required for specific reflex areas. There is, in fact, a particular head and sinuses technique which involves 'walking' the thumb of one hand down each of the toes on the opposite foot. There is another technique for the areas corresponding to the eyes and the ears and another for the neck and throat. However, diabetics, pregnant women, and anyone with specific disorders of the legs or feet or any acute or chronic illness, should always consult a qualified practitioner.

Finding A Practitioner

For a list of practitioners or further information write, sending a SAE to:

The British Reflexology Association, 12 Pond Road, London SE3 9JL.

Further Reading

Reflexology: Headway Lifeguides by Chris Stormer (Headway)
Reflexology & Colour Therapy Workbook by Pauline Wills
   (Element Books)

10

OSTEOPATHY, CHIROPRACTIC AND ALEXANDER TECHNIQUE: MANIPULATIVE RELIEF

Many headaches are the result of muscle tension in the neck, so we can see that osteopathic or chiropractic treatment of headaches and migraines may be extremely helpful.

Osteopathy

The practice of osteopathy is based on the theory that disorders are due to loss of structural integrity which can be restored by manipulation of the skeletal system.

The Origins And Theory Of Osteopathy

The father of Osteopathy, Andrew Taylor Still, was born in 1828 in Virginia, USA. He became disenchanted with then current medical practices after the deaths of his three children. Trained as an engineer, later as a physician, he practised medicine in the army. Applying the trained logic of an engineer, he reasoned that illness should be treated for its causes and not simply its symptoms. Still's studies of the interdependence of the body's structure (i.e. a trapped nerve in the shoulder may be the cause of pain in the wrist, for example) and his Christian beliefs (he was a minister's son) led him to conclude that the human body contained the ability to heal itself, and that the body must be viewed in its entirety, as a complete unit. Still's approach to medicine, then, was holistic. His theory of osteopathy (he coined the name himself) is based on three principles:

- the normal, healthy body has its own innate powers of healing and defence mechanisms;

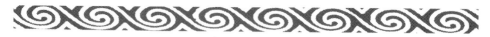

- the body is a unit and one malfunctioning part will have effects on other parts;
- the body is in its optimum state of operation when it has maximum structural mobility and flexibility.

On this last principle, Still has sometimes been misquoted and misunderstood. He did not mean that all disease stems from problems of the spine or of the skeleton as a whole. What he did mean was that the skeleton, as the body's structure, has a cause and effect relationship on the health of the rest of the body, its muscles, blood system and joints.

Osteopathy as a medical practice became widely accepted and practised in the USA and today its validity is recognised the world over.

A Modern Osteopath

Osteopathy, in Still's time, was used to cure any and all of the body's ills. Today, osteopathy confines itself to the treatment of problems of the spine, ligaments, muscles and bones. It promotes lymphatic drainage and improves breathing.

A visit to an osteopath begins with an examination of the problem area. The patient's posture and ease of mobility will be studied from the moment of entering the consulting room. The muscles, joints and the entire surface of the body are examined to reveal any problem areas which may need gentle correction. The osteopath does not aim to transform every patient's skeleton into a model of perfection – this would be medically impossible, in any case. An osteopath's aim is to correct, where necessary, any problems, because they are limiting the body's correct functioning.

Cranial Osteopathy

Cranial osteopathy was first explored by W G Sutherland, a pupil of Still. Sutherland's research showed that the skull's joints may play an important role in respiration and the central nervous system. Headaches, dizziness and nausea may well be the effect of problems in the skull – a bump on the head which you thought at the time was not serious could be the root cause of your present problem. Cranial osteopathy in this case may well be the answer.

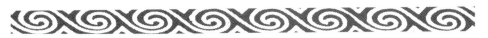

Osteopathy For A Healthy Life

Once an osteopath has set you on the road to healing, the lessons learned concerning correct posture and breathing can continue to be applied in daily life, keeping your body structure and health in good form.

Chiropractic

Chiropractic treats backache, neck pain and low backache by gentle manipulation of the spine. The theory is that since the spine has nerves radiating off it which reach every part of the body, the spine is the key to eliminating pain in the whole body. A displaced vertebra, for example, puts pressure on a nerve, which may result in pain in a limb or give rise to a headache. The chiropractor uses his/her skill to discover which vertebra is misaligned and then to correct it. No drugs are used, since chiropractic is entirely manipulative.

Usually people see a chiropractor for problems of the spine, joints or muscles. Since the whole nervous system is linked to the nerves from the spine, a chiropractor may help with problems of the nervous system.

An initial consultation with a chiropractor will feature an in-depth historical analysis to include childhood injuries and current lifestyle. Some chiropractors will also conduct a thorough physical examination, including a routine examination, similar to that which you would receive from a GP. A manipulative examination of the muscles, skin, bone and joints reveals to the chiropractor whether chiropractic is in fact suitable for your problem or if you should be referred back to your GP. The manipulative examination explores the texture, tenderness and movement of the body from which the chiropractor makes his/her diagnosis. For some chiropractors, X-rays may form part of the examination, but this is not the case with a McTimoney practitioner.

If chiropractic is called for, treatment techniques might include massage of the muscles and ligaments, stretching of ligaments, instruction on posture, rotary massage and direct localised pressure on the troubled body part. Depending on the scale of the medical problem, benefits may be apparent after only one session or after several.

Chiropractic, like osteopathy, is a manipulative therapy, and their

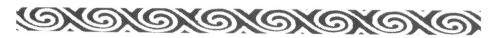

goals are therefore similar. However, osteopathy concentrates on the movement of the joints and uses leverage more than chiropractic, while chiropractic places emphasis on direct contact on the spine's vertebrae for their adjustment. Chiropractic works more on the spine and its effects on the nervous system and related effects on the rest of the body.

For headaches and migraine, the chiropractor will check the spine and then align the appropriate vertebrae. The basic chiropractic manipulation, usually known as *adjustment,* is a high velocity thrust. The speed and precision of the adjustments make the treatment relatively gentle.

The Alexander Technique

George Bernard Shaw, Aldous Huxley and Roald Dahl all used the Alexander Technique, as do John Cleese and Paul Newman. The Alexander Technique is highly valued by the acting profession for its lessons in breathing techniques, posture and movement. People find that adopting correct techniques in breathing and movement bring about psychological as well as physical changes, making them feel more confident, graceful and strong.

The Alexander Technique corrects any bad habits of poor posture, breathing and speech defects. It was evolved by F M Alexander, an Australian who died in 1955 at the age of 86. He evolved the technique because, as an aspiring actor, he was hampered by loss of voice while performing. After numerous consultations with doctors to no effect, he decided his problem lay within, and consequently began his observations of his posture and how it changed when he spoke. He discovered that he had a tendency to move his head back and down, which depressed his vocal cords and shortened his spine. Years of patient self-observation and analysis eventually retrained his habits and his speech problem was resolved. Actors of the day visited him to learn his techniques, and in time his acting career gave way to training students and future Alexander teachers.

This technique of attaining correct posture can help by reducing tensions that may have gone unnoticed for decades. The way we hold our heads can contribute, among other things, to headaches and even migraine.

Glynn Macdonald, a highly experienced teacher of the Alexander Technique and author of *Headway Lifeguides : Alexander Technique,* writes:

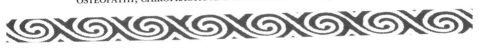

The Alexander Technique is about learning how this relationship of the head, neck and back works to maximise the body's potential. Alexander considered this postural understanding so important he called it the 'Primary Control'. 'Primary' means earliest, chief or most important; 'Control' means the power of directing or commanding, so this chief command is the most important part of our Directions for Use. Without an understanding of how this relationship works, we are limiting our whole physical potential, so let us look at how this Primary Control operates.

In all vertebrates, that is animals with backbones, and that includes us, the position of the head is very important. Where the head leads, the body will follow. It is like the engine of the train with the carriages following. The four-legged animals have it easier than us, as the direction of their head and back follows the same direction as their line of movement.

When it comes to human beings, this becomes more complicated. The principle is the same – where the head leads the body follows – but when we stood up the line of movement changed. We move forward but the direction along the spine has to continue up through the head.

The head is delicately balanced on the backbone, which is a column of vertebrae and discs. The head is a heavy mass, weighing between eight and fifteen pounds, with the ability to nod freely forward in a subtle, gentle movement. It is not meant to be fixed stiffly on to the spine, but often the neck muscles are so tight that this very important releasing movement cannot happen. A lot of distress in the form of headaches, shoulder and back pain is caused by the restriction of movement in the relationship between the head and neck.

Learning The Alexander Technique

There is a register of teachers of the Alexander Technique which you can consult. A teacher is really necessary to learn the technique correctly – the teacher will be able to observe your current movements and make you aware of any tensions which may need to be released. You can study the technique from books, but it is rather like learning to speak a foreign language; you can only achieve so much without direct contact.

Finding A Practitioner

For a list of practitioners or further information write, sending a SAE to:

Osteopathy
The General Council and Register of Osteopaths, 56 London Street, Reading, Berkshire RG14BQ;

The British Naturopathy and Osteopathy Association, 6 Netherall Gardens, London NW3 5RR;

Chiropractic

The British Chiropractic Association, 29 Whitley Street, Reading, Berkshire RG2 2EG;

The Institute of Pure Chiropractic, 14 Park End Street, Oxford OX2 1HH;

Alexander Technique

Society of Teachers of the Alexander Technique (STAT), 10 Station House, 266 Fulham Road, London SW10 9EL.

Further Reading

Alexander Technique: Headway Lifeguides by Glynn Macdonald (Headway)

Chiropractic by S Moore (Macdonald Optima)

Chiropractic Today by Copland-Griffiths (Thorsons)

Osteopathy Self Treatment by Leon Chaitow (Thorsons)

11

CONCLUSION

As a centre of perception and thinking, the head is the most sensitive alarm system of the body and when it aches it is sending a signal. As we have seen in the earlier chapters of this book, headaches can be caused by a wide variety of factors. Sometimes described as the 'silent cry of an over-burdened mind', a headache occurs when we strive too hard or develop an obsession with 'succeeding' and 'getting on in life'. Stress builds up and a tension headache follows. Pause for a moment and ask yourself: 'Is it worth pursuing never-ending targets, or should I let go of my stubbornness and pride to restore balance in myself?'

Maybe you have had these thoughts and emotions but suppressed them. When feelings and thoughts are suppressed and not given expression, they affect the head, as they have no outlet. Negative emotions can also cause headaches, as can a sense of self-doubt.

A headache, therefore, is not simply a matter of blood dilation or related problems, such as infection or indigestion. It is a classic example of a body–mind interaction. But then, which disorder is not?

Does it make a difference which of the therapies, orthodox or complementary, you choose to attain health and well-being? There is no simple answer to this. If you are looking to eliminate the symptoms of your disorder as opposed to healing, then any therapy that quickly and effectively deals with the symptoms would be acceptable. However, if you consider healing as regaining good health and being wholly well again, then you have to look at all the therapies in a very different light.

When the body malfunctions, it has an effect on us at various levels. If I say I have a headache, it means that the pain which is manifesting itself in my head is in me as a person . If I just treat the head by, for example, taking aspirin, it means I am disregarding the source of inner pain.

Neither the GP and his/her drugs, nor the herbalist and his/her herbs, nor the aromatherapist and his/her essential oils, nor the acupuncturist and his/her needles, nor the osteopath and his/her manipulation, nor the anthroposophical doctor with his/her art therapy, eurythmy and hydrotherapy can heal. **Only you can heal**

yourself. 'Each patient carries his own doctor inside him,' said Dr Albert Schweitzer.

In order to begin the process of healing, you must want to achieve health. The will to get better comes into play and mind–body interaction has to be acknowledged.

An understanding and acceptance of this body–mind interaction will result in an integration of the body and the mind in the process of achieving wellness. That is what healing is all about. If this is understood, then it is easy to understand why the therapies described in this book can be effective. Whatever therapy we may choose, it can only be effective if we have a positive attitude towards the healing technique and the person who helps us to heal ourselves.

The culture of dependency spawned by modern medical intervention, the emphasis on curing the sick parts of the body, has conditioned us to lose faith in our own ability to heal ourselves. We have come to rely on medication as a form of reassurance and believe that the prescription will 'cure'.

The root of this thinking is attributed to René Descartes whose dictum, 'I think therefore I am', crystallised the concept of separating *res cognitas* (the realm of the mind) and *res extensa* (the realm of matter). His perception of the material world has so permeated our culture that we now view the human body as an elaborate machine made up of assembled parts.

This legacy of dualism has guided and moulded the basis of modern medicine up to the present time.

Modern study of disease has focused on biological processes, attributing the causes of all illness to biological factors. Modern medicine, preoccupied with measurements, statistical models and double-blind crossover studies, fails to take into account the person as a whole and appears to preclude the human potential for self-healing. The mind–body relationship has been ignored in healing. Whatever the disease, unless we accept that this relationship does exist, it is not possible to achieve true healing or true health and well-being.

We must first recognise that mind and body are both aspects of the human whole; that they are interrelated and cannot be seen in isolation from each other. The state of perfect balance between mind and body, as experienced in childhood, can be achieved. To do that, we have to understand the role of the mind and the body working and affecting each other.

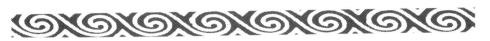

There is a complex system of information that conveys messages between the mind and the body contained in our bloodstream.

Regulation by the pituitary gland and the hypothalamus (a region of the brain situated between the eyes which has nerve connections from all over the nervous system) controls the psychological and emotional activity in relation to the physical function of the body. A good example of such a connection is the vegus nerve which links the stomach to the hypothalamus, with the result that stress or anxiety can cause stomach upsets.

We have seen that the immune system is indispensable for defence against disease-causing substances. However, we can be left vulnerable to disease if certain hormones are released by the adrenal glands which disrupt the relationship between the brain and the immune system. In addition to stress, this disruption can be caused by repressed feelings such as prolonged anger, bitterness and other negative emotions and thoughts.

The *limbic system*, a ring shaped area in the brain, consists of clusters of nerve cells, including the hypothalamus. Called the 'seat of emotions', the limbic system regulates very basic nervous functions, such as sweating, digestion and heart rate, and has a bearing on our emotions and sense of smell. The limbic system is therefore important in the body-mind relationship. This, in turn, is influenced by the cerebral cortex (the part of the brain responsible for thinking, perception, memory and all other intellectual activity). Stress is an example of the result of the alarm bells sounded by the cerebral cortex when it perceives a life-threatening situation. As soon as the alarm bells ring, the limbic system and consequently the nervous system and the immune system are all galvanised into action. The reaction is tense muscles, constricted blood vessels and other symptoms that set into motion a general nervous disarray. Some reactions are instantaneous, such as blushing when your emotions produce the effect of blood rushing to your face; others, such as repressed anger, are cumulative and take longer to manifest themselves in the form of disease.

There is little doubt that there is an innate link between the mind and the body, each affecting the other. Negative thoughts and emotions will result in weakened defences which will lead to disease and, ultimately, death. Our recognition of the body–mind connection is reflected in our everyday language when we say, 'he is eaten up with jealousy', or 'his heart is broken', or 'the stress is killing him', or 'he is worn down with grief', or 'she is radiantly happy'.

Most of the traditional healing disciplines, based on different world views and cosmological principles, all have a common thread: they deal with illness by considering human beings in the context of their relationship with the cosmos.

Human existence is not simply matter to which life has been added but rather is part of a complex energy structure. This basic fact is recognised in many medical cultures. Muslim physicians consider man as a psychosomatic unity endowed with a self-directing, purpose or vital force (*ruh*). The Yogic view is that the human body is is composed of three different manifestations, namely, the physical body (composed of flesh, blood and bone), the subtle body (containing the life force *prana*) and the spiritual body (which encompasses universal wisdom).

To the Hawaiians, health means energy. Good health is a state of *ehuehu* (abundant energy) and poor health is *pake* (weakness). Illness is caused by *mai* (tension) and healing is equated to the restoration of *lapau* (energy). Health therefore is a state of harmonious energy.

The American Indians think that Earth is a living organism, and that all creations on this earth contain a life force which are part of a harmonious whole. Illness occurs when this balance is upset and the purpose of healing ceremonies is to restore both personal and universal harmony.

Tai Chi is the Chinese way of increasing the energy flow in the body and strengthening the body's resistance to ward off disease. Tai Chi is thought to stimulate the kidney (seen as the life force energy) and to maintain vitality of mind, body and spirit.

Rudolf Steiner, the founder of anthroposophy, sought to go beyond the idea of healing the body. His acute perception led him to explore the spiritual side of existence, which led to an understanding of the ways of stimulating the natural healing forces in the person. Healing was a matter of considering the interrelation between the four aspects of the human being (physical body, etheric body, astral body and the ego) and treating them as a whole.

There are striking similarities in the various healing systems reviewed above. Call it by any name – prana, chi, life force, ehuehu, etheric energy – we all have it in us. It is up to the 'doctor inside', to borrow Albert Schweitzer's phrase, to harness this healing force within us and so to achieve that state of balance between body, mind and spirit.

Of late, the holistic model of health-care has begun to gain

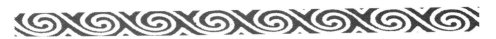

momentum. The proponents of this model have gone some way to counter some of the overly mechanistic and reductionist streaks in modern medicine, although this does not mean denying the undoubted achievements of science. Holism is based on the premise that the human organism is a multidimensional being, possessing body, mind and spirit, all inextricably linked, and that disease results from an imbalance, either from within or from an external force. The human body possesses a powerful and innate capacity to heal itself by bringing itself back into a state of balance, and so the primary task of the practitioner is to encourage and assist the body in its attempts to heal itself. The practitioner's role is that of an educator rather than an interventionist. If patients see themselves as self-healing agents, they will naturally want to exercise their own power and be in control of their own health.

The true test of healing must surely be a practical manifestation of harmony between the mind, the body and the spirit. Holism has some answers, but matters of the spirit, while acknowledged, remain untouched and are sometimes even avoided in practice. Yet without the spiritual dimension, no system of healing can be truly whole. There can be no true self-healing and no true holistic medicine unless the spirit is also recognised.

You picked up this book because you suffer from headaches or migraine and because you have an open mind – you are willing to explore different types of interaction between the body and the mind. **You** are responsible for drawing spirit into the equation and the final message of this book is that so-called 'holism' that looks only at the mind and the body, ignoring the spirit is an illusion – go for a truer reality and use this book as, perhaps, a first step on the road to uniting body, mind and spirit.

GLOSSARY

Acute Symptom that comes on suddenly, usually for a short period.

Adrenaline Hormone released by the adrenal gland, triggered by fear or stress.

Allergy A condition caused by the reaction of the immune system to a specific substance.

Allopathy A term used to describe conventional drug-based medicine.

Amino acids A group of chemical compounds containing nitrogen that form the basic building blocks in the production of protein. Of the 22 known amino acids, 8 are considered essential because they cannot be made by the body and therefore must be obtained from the diet.

Anaemia A condition that results when there is a low level of red blood cells.

Analgesic A substance that relieves pain.

Antibiotic A medication that helps to treat infection caused by bacteria.

Antibody Protein molecule released by the body's immune system that neutralises or counteracts foreign organisms *(antigen)*.

Antidote A substance that neutralizes or counteracts the effects of a poison.

Antigen Any substance that can trigger the immune system to release an antibody to defend the body against infection and disease. When harmless substances like pollen are mistaken for harmful antigens by the immune system, allergy results.

Antihistamine A chemical that counteracts the effects of histamine, a chemical released during allergic reactions.

Antioxidants Substances which inhibit oxidation by destroying free radicals. Common antioxidants are vitamins A, C, E and the minerals selenium and zinc.

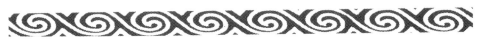

Antiseptic A preparation which has the ability to destroy undesirable micro-organisms.

Atopy A predisposition to various allergic conditions like asthma, hay fever, urticaria and eczema.

Auto-immune disease A condition in which the immune system attacks the body's own tissue e.g. rheumatoid arthritis.

Beta carotene A plant substance which can be converted into vitamin A.

Cartilage Connective tissue that forms part of the skeletal system, such as the joints.

Chi Chinese term for the energy that circulates through the meridians.

Cholesterol A fat compound, manufactured in the body, that facilitates the transportation of fat in the blood stream.

Chronic A disorder that persists for a long time; in contrast to acute.

Collagen Main component of the connective tissue.

Constitutional treatment Treatment determined by an assessment of a person's physical, mental and emotional states.

Contagious A term referring to a disease that can be transferred from one person to another by direct contact.

Corticosteroid Drugs used to treat inflammation similar to corticosteroid hormones produced by the adrenal glands that control the body's use of nutrients and excretion of salts and water in urine.

Detoxification Treatment to eliminate or reduce poisonous substances *(toxins)* from the body.

Diuretic Substance that increases urine flow.

DNA A molecule carrying genetic information in most organisms.

Elimination diet A diet which eliminates allergic foods.

Endorphins Substances which have the property of suppressing pain. They are also involved in controlling the body's response to stress.

Enkephalins Protein molecules which have an analgesic (painkilling) effect as well as producing a sedative effect.

Enzyme A protein catalyst that speeds chemical reactions in the body.

Essential fatty acids Substances that cannot be made by the body and therefore need to be obtained from the diet.

Essential oil Highly fragrant essence extracted from a plant by distillation. A liquid present in plants in tiny droplets.

Free radicals Highly unstable atoms or group of atoms containing at least one unpaired electron.

Histamine A chemical released during an allergic reaction, responsible for redness and swelling that occur in inflammation.

Holistic medicine Any form of therapy aimed at treating the whole person – mind, body and spirit.

Iridology The science of diagnosis by observing the iris of the eye.

Lymphocyte A type of white blood cell found in lymph nodes. Some lymphocytes are important in the immune system.

Malignant A term that describes a condition that gets progressively worse, resulting in death.

Meridian Energy pathways that connect the acupuncture and acupressure points and the internal organs.

Mucous membrane Pink tissue that lines most cavities and tubes in the body, such as the mouth, nose etc.

Mucus The thick fluid secreted by the mucous membranes.

Neurotransmitter A chemical that transmits nerve impulses between nerve cells.

Oxidation Chemical process of combining with oxygen or of removing hydrogen.

Placebo A chemically inactive substance given instead of a drug, often used to compare the efficacy of medicines in clinical trials.

Platelets Cells responsible for repairing breaches in the lining of the blood vessels.

Potency A term used in homoeopathy to describe the number of times a substance has been diluted.

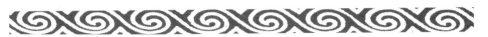

Prostaglandin Hormone-like compounds manufactured from essential fatty acids.

Rotation diet A diet that ensures that a person eats each food once every few days (minimum 4 days) as opposed to having a few foods that are consumed regularly.

Sclerosis Process of hardening or scarring.

Stimulant A substance that increases energy.

Toxin A poisonous protein produced by disease-causing bacteria.

Vaccine A preparation given to induce immunity against a specific infectious disease.

Vasoconstriction A term used to describe the constriction of blood vessels.

Vasodilation A term used to describe the dilation of blood vessels.

Vitamin Essential nutrient that the body needs to act as a catalyst in normal processes of the body.

Withdrawal Termination of a habit-forming substance.

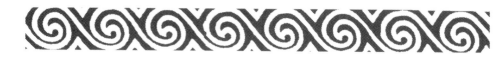

INDEX

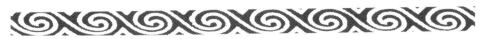

THE NATURAL MEDICINES SOCIETY

The Natural Medicines Society is a registered charity representing the consumer voice for freedom of choice in medicine. The Society needs the support of every individual who uses natural medicines and who is concerned about their continued existence in order to achieve the necessary changes needed to accomplish their wider availability and acceptance within the NHS.

The Society's aims are to improve the standing and practice of natural medicine by encouraging education and research, and by co-operating with the government and the EC on their registration, safety and efficacy. A major drawback in this work has been that none of the Department of Health's licensing bodies has any experts from these systems of medicine sitting on their committees – this has meant that not one of the natural medicines assessed by them has been judged by anyone with an understanding of the therapy's practice. Since the formation of the Society, it has worked towards the establishment of expert representation on the committees appraising these medicines.

To fulfil these aims, the NMS formed the Medicines Advisory Research Committee in February 1988. Known as MARC, its members are doctors, practitioners, pharmacists and other experts in natural medicines. It is the members of MARC who undertake much of the necessary technical and legal work. They have discussed and submitted proposals to the Department of Health's Medicines Control Agency (MCA), on how the EC Directive for Homoeopathic Medicinal Products can be incorporated into the existing UK system, and how medicines outside the orthodox range can be fairly evaluated.

The EC Directive for Homoeopathic Medicinal Products was eventually passed as European law in September 1992, incorporating anthroposophical and biochemic medicines, as well as homoeopathic. With discussions regarding the implementation of

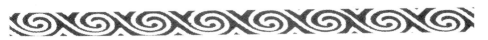

the Homoeopathic Directive now in progress, the MARC's work begins in earnest.

In July 1993, the MCA sent out their consultation paper regarding the implementation of the Directive, which incorporates many of the suggestions submitted by MARC. In it they propose to set up a committee of experts to advise on the registration of homoeopathic, anthroposophic and biochemic medicines. This is a major step forward for the Society, and homoeopathy in general.

With MARC members becoming increasingly involved in the legislative process of the implementation of the Directive, the Natural Medicines Society can now move forward from the short-term aim of protecting the availability of the medicines, to the longer-term aims of promoting and developing their usage and status by instigating and supporting research and education. The NMS has already sponsored some research – it is important to stress here that the Society does not endorse, support or condone animal experimentation – including an expedition to the rain forests in search of medicinal plants, supporting a cancer research project at the Royal London Homoeopathic Hospital and contributing to a methodology Research Fellowship. On the educational side, the Society has published two booklets, with several more planned and has co-sponsored a seminar for doctors and medical students.

The Natural Medicines Society depends upon its membership to continue this unique and important work – please add your support by joining us.

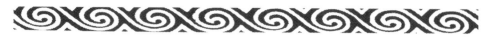

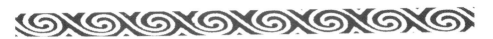

IF YOU ARE NOT ALREADY A MEMBER
WHY NOT JOIN THE
NATURAL MEDICINES SOCIETY?

(BLOCK CAPITALS PLEASE)

Mr/Mrs/Miss/Ms _____

Address _____

_____

Postcode _____ Tel. No. _____

There is no 'fixed' annual membership fee. Please indicate below the amount you wish to pay: minimum £5 (students and unwaged); European countries £15; non-EC £20.

£5 _____ £10 _____ £15 _____

N.B. Pay by Deed of Covenant and/or Direct Debit if you can—please ask for details.

Donations and offers of practical help are also always welcome to aid our fight to return natural medicines to the mainstream of medical practice.

I enclose a donation of £ _____

Please return this form with your remittance (cheques and PO's payable to The Natural Medicines Society), to:

THE NMS MEMBERSHIP OFFICE,
EDITH LEWIS HOUSE,
ILKESTON,
DERBYS,
DE7 8EJ.

(Registered charity no.327468)

You will receive your Membership Card, Member's Handbook, Quarterly Newsletter.

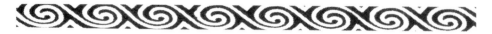

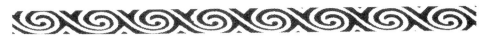

Author Profiles

Hasnain Walji is a writer and freelance journalist specialising in health, nutrition and complementary therapies, with a special interest in dietary supplementation. A contributor to several journals on environmental and Third World consumer issues, he was the founder and editor of *The Vitamin Connection – An International Journal of Nutrition, Health and Fitness,* published in the UK, Canada and Australia, focusing on the link between health and diet. He also launched Healthy Eating, a consumer magazine focusing on the concept of a well-balanced diet, and has written a script for a six-part television series, *The World of Vitamins,* shortly to be produced by a Danish Television company. His latest book, *The Vitamin Guide- Essential Nutrients for Healthy Living,* has just been published, and he is currently involved in developing NutriPlus™: a nutrition database and diet analysis programme for an American software development company.

Dr Andrea Kingston MB ChB, DRCOG, MRCGP, DCH is a Buckinghamshire GP in a five-doctor training practice who has for some years been interested in complementary approaches to healthcare as well as psychiatry and Neuro-linguistic Programming. Hypnotherapy is her major interest, and she has used this technique to help patients throughout the last eight years. As a company doctor to Volkswagen Audi, she contributes regular articles to the company magazine, *Link.* In the past, she has served as a member of the Family Practitioners Committee and as the President of the Milton Keynes Medical Society.

Books by the same authors in the Headway Healthwise series:

- Skin Conditions
- Asthma & Hay Fever
- Alcoholism, Smoking & Tranquillisers
- Heart Health
- Arthritis & Rheumatism

Headway

Your Health in Your Hands

HEADWAY LIFEGUIDES

Simple and practical introductions to complementary
therapies for the complete beginner.

Tai Chi
0 340 60008 X
£8.99

Alexander Technique
0 340 59680 5
£8.99

Herbalism
0 340 56575 6 £7.99

Aromatherapy
0 340 55950 0 £7.99

Homoeopathy
0 340 56578 0 £7.99

Massage
0 340 55949 7 £7.99

Reflexology
0 340 55594 7 £7.99

Shiatsu
0 340 55321 9 £7.99

Yoga
0 340 55948 9 £7.99

PUBLISHING SEPTEMBER 1994

Visualisation
0 340 61107 3
£6.99

Acupressure
0 340 61106 5
£6.99

HEADWAY HEALTHWISE

Self-help guides to managing common problems
using integrated complementary and orthodox
approaches. Endorsed by The Natural
Medicines Society.

NEW SERIES

Asthma and Hay Fever
0 340 60558 8

Skin Conditions
0 340 60559 6

Alcohol, Smoking,
Tranquillisers
0 340 60561 8

Headaches and
Migraines
0 340 60560 X

Arthritis and
Rheumatism
0 340 60563 4

Heart Health
0 340 60562 6

£6.99 each

Headway is an imprint of

Hodder & Stoughton
A MEMBER OF THE HODDER HEADLINE GROUP